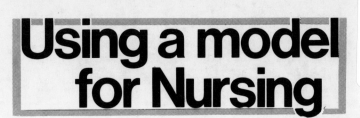

Using a model for Nursing

NANCY ROPER is the author of *Principles of Nursing, Man's Anatomy, Physiology, Health and Environment* and the *Churchill Livingstone Nurses Dictionary*. She trained at the General Infirmary in Leeds and later spent 15 years at the Cumberland Infirmary School of Nursing as Principal Tutor. In 1970, following a period of full-time writing, she was awarded a research fellowship from the Commonwealth Nurses' War Memorial Fund. The research, into clinical experience in nurse education, was undertaken from the Nursing Research Unit at the University of Edinburgh and gained the MPhil degree. From 1975 to 1978 she was Nursing Officer (Research) at the Scottish Home and Health Department.

WIN LOGAN is Head of Department of Health and Nursing Studies, Glasgow College of Technology, Scotland. She was Executive Director of the International Council of Nurses (ICN) from 1978–80. She had already gained considerable knowledge and experience of nursing internationally, having worked or served as a consultant in Canada, the USA, Malaysia and Iraq. In 1971–72 she acted as Chief Nursing Officer at the newly created Ministry of Health in Abu Dhabi. Prior to moving to the ICN she worked for 4 years at the Scottish Home and Health Department where she had responsibility for nursing education. She took to that post experience gained from a 12-year term of office, first as lecturer and latterly as senior lecturer, in the Department of Nursing Studies at the University of Edinburgh. She is an arts graduate of that university and did her basic nurse education at the Royal Infirmary of Edinburgh.

ALISON TIERNEY is a graduate nurse and was one of the first nurses in the UK to gain a doctoral degree. Her PhD was obtained for research done in the field of mental handicap nursing while holding a Nursing Research Fellowship awarded by the Scottish Home and Health Department. From 1973–80 she was a lecturer in the Department of Nursing Studies at the University of Edinburgh. Amongst other things, this post involved her in the development of the foundation nursing course for first-year students and in the clinical supervision of students at various stages in the degree/nursing programme. During 1976 and 1977 she acted as nurse adviser to the Edinburgh Medical Group research project, set up to develop methods of studying medical ethics and moral issues in health care.

Nancy Roper, Win Logan and Alison Tierney are the joint authors of *The Elements of Nursing* and *Learning to Use the Process of Nursing*.

Using a model for Nursing

EDITED BY

NANCY ROPER
MPhil RGN RSCN RNT

WINIFRED W. LOGAN
MA DNS(Educ) RGN RNT

ALISON J. TIERNEY
BSc(Soc Sc—Nurs) PhD RGN

CHURCHILL LIVINGSTONE
EDINBURGH LONDON MELBOURNE AND NEW YORK 1983

CHURCHILL LIVINGSTONE
Medical Division of Longman Group UK Limited

Distributed in the United States of America by Churchill Livingstone Inc.,
1560 Broadway, New York, N. Y. 10036, and by associated companies,
branches and representatives throughout the world.

First published 1983
  Reprinted 1984
  Reprinted 1988
  Reprinted 1990

ISBN 0-443-02676-9

British Library Cataloguing in Publication Data
Using a model for nursing.
  1. Nursing
  I. Roper, Nancy   II. Logan, Winifred W.
  III. Tierney, Alison J.
  610.73   RT41

Library of Congress Cataloging in Publication Data
Main entry under title:
Using a model for nursing.
  1. Nursing. I. Roper, Nancy,
II. Logan, Winifred W. III. Tierney, Alison J.
[DNLM: 1. Nursing care. 2. Nursing process.
3. Models, Theoretical. WY 100 U85]
RT41.U84 1983   610.73   82-14656

Produced by Longman Singapore Publishers Pte Ltd
Printed in Singapore

Preface

This book is the third in a trilogy. In our first book *The Elements of Nursing* (1980) we describe a model for nursing which has as its focus twelve activities of living (ALs), and the model incorporates the process of nursing. Nursing is viewed as helping patients to solve, alleviate, cope with, or prevent problems related to activities of living rather than as treating patients with specific disease conditions — the approach implicit in a 'disease' model. A crucial point about this concept is that it includes for each patient/client an individual approach.

In our second book *Learning to Use the Process of Nursing* (1981) we describe how this way of thinking about nursing can be applied in practice within the framework of our model for nursing. The book contains a series of presentations which exemplify a particular aspect of application, and each has as its focus a particular patient. The patients presented are not 'real' but they are realistic and they represent the kinds of patients which nurse learners encounter even in their early clinical experience. In retrospect, the second book is a crucial link between the first and third books.

This third book describes a project set up to test our belief that the model is a conceptual framework which can be used in any health care setting. The project involves real patients and the nursing studies were carried out and written by practising nurses. So this third book is different from its predecessors; it is an edited publication. Hereafter in this text, therefore, we refer to ourselves as editors.

In the first chapter we describe the project, and the second chapter gives a brief outline of the model for nursing. The main body of the book, however, consists of nine chapters each of which is contributed by nurses selected from a variety of health care settings who are directly involved in nursing patients/clients and who agreed to use the model, which incorporates the process, while nursing one patient/client. Each chapter, therefore, describes how the contributors tackled this assignment and they offer comments on the use of the model as a conceptual framework for nursing. In the final chapter we discuss the nine contributions and, in the light of the project, offer our reflections on the model for nursing.

From such a limited exercise it is not possible to draw firm conclusions. Nevertheless, important points have emerged which will be of interest to all nurses who are concerned about individualising nursing, whatever the clinical setting. In particular it will be useful for students who require a conceptual framework and a mode of thinking to help them to learn about nursing and how nursing data can be documented.

We consider this publication to be unique in its collaboration between nurse authors and nurse practitioners and an important development in linking theory and practice.

We wish to thank the publishers for participating in this venture; the contributors who worked hard and long; and the nursing staff in various hospital and community settings for their co-operation and understanding while the project was carried out. For ourselves we consider that the effort has been well worthwhile. We hope readers will find useful ideas in the studies and in the conclusions which will stimulate further thinking about nursing. If the practice of nursing is to be congruent with reality, the documentation must be practical for nurses to use, yet comprehensive in giving a profile of the patient as a person. We consider this book to be a step in that direction.

Edinburgh 1983   NR, WL, AT

Contributors

Chapter 3

Annina B. Mayhew BA RGN SCM RNT
Nurse teacher

Elizabeth Y. Howie BSc(Soc Sc—Nurs) RGN SCM NDN
Sister, Diabetic Clinic

Chapter 4

Elizabeth M. Stewart BSc(Soc Sc) RGN SCM RNT
Lecturer in nursing studies

Heather C. Strachan
Student nurse

Chapter 5

Effie P. Alexander RGN SCM HVCert FWT
Health visitor

Chapter 6

Euphemia M. Taylor RGN SCM Midwife Clinical
Instructor's Certificate
Clinical teacher (Midwifery)

Molly Coventry RGN SCM RNT BA
Director of Nurse Education

Chapter 7

Irene Reid RGN
Ward sister

Anne Blackie RGN RSCN
Ward sister

Chapter 8

Mary Birkett Colquhoun BSc(Soc Sc—Nurs) RGN
RSCN NDN
Ward sister

Agnes Fraser BSc(Soc Sc—Nurs) RGN NDN
Staff nurse

Chapter 9

Niall Grant RMN
Staff nurse

Bernard White RMN SRN RGN RNT
Nurse tutor

Chapter 10

Mary Cooke RGN SCM NDN
District nurse

Sheila Moir RGN SCM RSCN QIDNS HV DNT RNT
Lecturer in nursing studies

Chapter 11

Marjorie Armstrong SRN
Sister, Neurosurgical ward

Anne Jarvie RGN SCM
Senior Nursing Officer

Contents

Note
The studies described in this book involved the participation of patients/clients in the hospital and home settings. Before an individual study proceeded, patient/client permission was invited and obtained. Pseudonyms and fictional geographical data are used in the text to protect the identity of the patients/clients. Dates of birth have been deliberately omitted.

Illustrations
In addition to the Roper, Logan and Tierney Patient Assessment Forms, other forms were used by contributors. The following forms were already in use in the contributors' hospitals or working environment: Figs 3.5, 3.6, 5.2, 5.3, 7.1, 7.2, 9.4 and 10.7.

All other forms were designed by the contributors prior to and during their participation in this study.

1 Introduction

At international level, the World Health Organization is helping member governments to think and act in terms of what is now a well-known catch phrase: 'Health for all by the year 2000' and the International Council of Nurses is emphasising nursing's contribution to this approach. At national level, various statutory bodies are proposing basic education programmes for nurses which put more emphasis on prevention of disease, and are advocating a health model rather than a disease model for nursing. At local level there is an increasing awareness that health and disease are closely related to life-style and activities of living. So, although for about two decades, some individuals and groups have been avant garde in advocating this 'health' approach, there is now much more general acceptance of the need for nursing to loosen its attachment to the 'disease' model which has been in the ascendancy in many countries of the world throughout this century.

Over the last ten years too, much has been written and said about the process of nursing. But now some basic programmes are incorporating this mode of thinking in their curriculum design. It is a logical way of thinking about any activity so it is not surprising that it can be seen by many nurses as acceptable — assessing, planning, implementing and evaluating nursing. However, a mode of thinking does not exist in vacuo; there must be some conceptual framework within which it can be used. Perhaps indeed some of the difficulties experienced up till now in using the process stem from the lack of a model to give it relevance.

The editors of this book are suggesting their model for nursing as a relevant framework and the process of nursing as a mode of thinking. We are not inferring that this is the only conceptual framework; several other models have been suggested mainly by nurses in North America and it is stimulating to consider the different approaches. Of course a model, any model, must be a reflection of the real world and it is only of use if it assists thinking and action in the real world. If not, it is merely an academic exercise, interesting though that may be.

This book is about the real world of nursing. It is perhaps unique in that the main part has been written by practising nurses using the Roper, Logan and Tierney model for nursing; the book is not a publication by armchair academics. It involves nurses writing about the nursing they do every day and writing about it for other nurses. Indeed the content of the nine main chapters is presented largely as it was submitted with minimum editorial change. Readers are invited to abstract from these chapters what is relevant and useful to the circumstances of their own everyday work.

BACKGROUND TO THE PROJECT

Even after writing the first two books (*The Elements of Nursing* and *Learning to Use the Process of Nursing*) we did not feel completely satisfied that our model was applicable to the real world of nursing. A logical way of testing the model's viability, we thought, would be to invite practising nurses to use the model, take note of any difficulties as they attempted to adopt this framework for nursing, then document the whole exercise. But could nurses be found who would be willing to accept such an undertaking? And if so, how many? And how many patients/clients would they be asked to nurse using this approach? And where would these nursing studies be carried out?

SELECTING THE NURSING SETTINGS

In *The Elements of Nursing* it was suggested that our model could be used in a variety of settings so we decided that practising nurses should be selected in a number of different practice areas. The model also includes the idea of a life-span, so we decided that there should be examples which would include patients/clients over an age range from infancy to old age. And in addition the model contains the idea that actual and potential problems can place a person anywhere along a continuum from total dependence to total independence so the examples were to include patients/clients at different points along the dependence/independence continuum.

After a great deal of thought it was decided that the settings should portray district nursing, health visiting, midwifery, an outpatient department, and nursing in medical, surgical, neurosurgical, geriatric, psychiatric and mental handicap wards. As a result of pressure of work which had not been anticipated the nurse in the mental handicap ward had to discontinue the study and at that time it was too late in the exercise to find a replacement. So the main part of the book contains accounts of the use of the model incorporating the process of nursing for one patient in each of nine settings.

The nine settings were chosen in two different Health Boards and the Chief Area Nursing Officers and other staff had to be informed about the activity for purposes of communication, and as a matter of courtesy. Co-operation was readily given and much interest was shown by many nursing and medical staff, especially those in direct contact with the contributors in their place of work.

SELECTING THE CONTRIBUTORS

The next step was to find the contributors. What sort of participation could we reasonably expect from busy practising nurses? In the first place to try it out, they would have to be conversant with the model, and how could we ensure this? It was decided that we would ask the contributors to read *The Elements of Nursing* as background preparation so that they would be familiar with the model and the twelve activities of living before commencing their nursing study.

Then the editors had to decide how much direct guidance should be given about how to tackle the assignment. Eventually it was agreed that the contributors should use the Patient Assessment Form presented in *The Elements of Nursing*; it reflects the components of the model, and the assessment stage of the process to the point of identifying actual and potential problems. Thereafter, however, very little guidance was given. This was deliberate. We wanted the contributors to have complete freedom to develop their own style of documentation for the three other stages of the process of nursing.

Obviously the tasks involved — the collection of data for the Patient Assessment Form; statement of goals; recording nursing interventions to achieve these goals; evaluation of whether or not the goals were achieved — would have to be done over and above the methods currently used in the ward or community setting where each contributor was working. So we would have to select contributors who had sufficient confidence in their professional expertise and sufficient individuality to think through their actions, analyse their actions and reactions, then write about the experience. It

would demand a considerable amount of commitment and tenacity of purpose.

Contrary to our initial apprehension, it was not at all difficult to find potential contributors. As it turned out almost all who were approached had some knowledge of the process of nursing although most were not conversant with our model. There was considerable enthusiasm for the project which was now beginning to take shape, despite acknowledged difficulties which might be encountered in undertaking the assignment and in committing to paper their difficulties and reflections.

Apart from the health visitor, the contributors worked in pairs and the following list gives some idea of the range of nursing staff who participated in the project:

Study	Contributors
A study of a diabetic patient	teacher
	sister
A study in a surgical ward	student
	lecturer
A health visitor's study of a mother and baby	health visitor
A midwife's study of a mother and baby	clinical teacher
	director of nurse education
A study of an elderly patient in hospital	ward sister
	ward sister
A study in a medical ward	ward sister
	staff nurse
A study in a psychiatric ward	staff nurse
	teacher
A district nursing study	district nurse
	lecturer
A study in a neurosurgical ward	sister
	senior nursing officer

And they all pay tribute to the colleagues at their place of work because without their co-operation and understanding, the collection of data would have been much more problematic.

It is not difficult to pick out the individuality and imaginative approaches used by the various contributors; these are apparent from the nine chapters and are discussed in some detail in the final chapter.

SELECTING THE PATIENTS/CLIENTS

Of course, the editors did not have control over the availability of patients/clients. Nevertheless an attempt was made to ensure that some of the patients selected by the contributors for the nursing studies would be male and some female; there would be a spread in age group; there would be a range in dependence/independence; and there would be flexibility regarding the period of data collection but it would not exceed six weeks. The actual choice of patient/client was left to the contributors because only they could assess the many factors which had to be taken into account. In most instances, the patient was newly referred to the hospital or community service.

It was agreed before the study commenced that each patient/client and his family would be informed and their permission invited and obtained, before proceeding with the study. Pseudonyms and fictional geographical data are used in the text to protect the identity of the patients/clients.

SHARING EXPERIENCE AND INFORMATION

So that the various contributors could meet each other, and meet the publisher and the three editors, an initial planning meeting of the invited contributors was arranged. The model for nursing was outlined; there was discussion about communication with nurse colleagues; about patient choice; about patient co-operation and permission; and a schedule for submission of material was drawn up and agreed. It was hoped that the whole exercise would be interesting and stimulating; but it was also a business arrangement so the written contracts with the publisher were explained and each contributor was given a copy of *The Elements of Nursing* which was to be used for reference. Each contributor was then assigned to one of the three editors as a liaison if any guidance were required and in fact, these informal discussions were a very rewarding aspect of the undertaking. As it happened some had considerable contact while planning and drafting their chapter; others minimal. In any event, editing has virtually consisted of clarification of a few points, and the data are presented as the contributors chose to document them.

The group met on a second occasion to report progress and share anxieties, for example about using some of the AL categories, about difficulties with the design of documents and about recording succinctly the nursing intervention. However, these were positive reactions and there was a marked mood of enthusiasm. It appeared that the colleagues of several contributors were also showing great interest in the project and

this was reassuring. Then at a later date we collected all the written material for co-ordination before reviewing the outcome of the project and writing the final chapter.

FOCUS ON THE PATIENT/CLIENT

Looking at the nine contributed chapters the reader may be tempted to comment that more should have been written in the text about the nine patients/clients as people; it is customary for this to be done in published patient studies. In fact, in all instances the patients were treated very much as individuals, and as individuals with a home and family and outside interests. However, for the purposes of this exercise, the text was used by the contributors to give an account of the thinking which went into the nursing of the patient, and to discuss the documentation of assessment, planning, implementation and evaluation. It is in the documentation accompanying the text that the individuality of the patients/clients and their life-styles are clearly reflected. This information is presented in a brief, concise style and the essence of good documentation is its succinctness. There is no inference that the presentation could not be improved, but it is hoped that the readers will use what is offered as growth points for perfecting their own form and style of documenting data.

In legal terms, documentation in nursing is becoming increasingly important and it is necessary to have accurate records of nursing practice. In professional terms, however, we must have useful documentation of data, not only for day-to-day effectiveness but also to build up a body of knowledge as a basis for nursing practice.

Before going on to the main section of the book where the contributors describe how they tackled the project and documented the nursing, Chapter 2 will describe the model for nursing and introduce the Patient Assessment Form. Chapter 2 is made up of material from *The Elements of Nursing* and *Learning to Use the Process of Nursing*.

REFERENCES

Roper N, Logan W W, Tierney A J 1980 The elements of nursing. Churchill Livingstone, Edinburgh

Roper N, Logan W W, Tierney A J 1981 Learning to use the process of nursing. Churchill Livingstone, Edinburgh

2

The model for nursing and its application

It is important to establish that the word 'model' was not used by the authors of *The Elements of Nursing* because it is an 'in' word. We sincerely believe that a model is useful in any discipline and this is no less true of nursing. A model seeks to embody the complexities of the subject, within its conceptual framework, and this cannot be achieved completely in a visual representation. The creators of a model have often devoted a lifetime to thinking about the subject before they write about their model. And it is the written word which describes the complexities of the subject encapsulated in the conceptual framework. The visual representation is merely a map or a prompt to the model. Models as conceived by their authors have to be understood before they can begin to influence practice, and the author's terminology has to be respected and used.

The model for nursing was first presented in a research monograph written by one of the editors (Roper, 1976). It is developed from a 'model of living' and both models have as their focus a set of 'activities of living'. In *The Elements of Nursing*, the model for nursing is described in Chapter 6 and the model of living on which it is based, in Chapter 2. The twelve ALs are discussed in Chapters 7 to 18. However, as a reminder to readers an outline of the two models is given below, because the contributors to this book were asked specifically to undertake a patient study using the Roper, Logan and Tierney model for nursing as their conceptual framework.

The model of living

What exactly are 'activities of living'? Most people could compose a list of everyday activities which they carry out in the process of living, and without doubt there would be common items in the lists. Probably most would mention eating, working, sleeping, washing and dressing as activities regularly carried out. If prompted, they would agree that breathing, communicating, eliminating and controlling body temperature are also essential activities, even if they are hardly aware of performing them. All of these, and others — such as mobilising, maintaining a safe environment, working and playing, expressing sexuality and dying — collectively contribute to the complex process of living. They are *activities of living*.

ACTIVITIES OF LIVING

The term 'activity of living' (AL) is used in this book as an all-embracing one. Each 'activity' has many dimensions, indeed it could be thought of as an overall activity composed of many particular activities.

The more one analyses the activities of living the more one realises just how complex each one of them is. Compounding this complexity is the fact that they are so interrelated. If the AL of maintaining a safe environment is neglected, accidents can happen and disability or untimely death may ensue. Communicating permeates several of the others: just imagine eating and drinking, working and playing, and expressing sexuality without communicating! And breathing is essential for all the ALs. So only for the purposes of description can they be separated and here only a brief description of each AL is necessary as an introduction to this mode of thinking about living.

Maintaining a safe environment

It is easy to think of safety in emergency situations. It may be less easy for people to think that many of the everyday activities are aimed at maintaining a safe environment. For example the home environment is kept safe by not leaving things lying about over which others could stumble; by keeping poisonous substances and dangerous articles in a safe place; by unplugging electric appliances at night; by guarding fires; and so on. Activities to achieve personal and domestic cleanliness aim at decreasing the number of micro-organisms in the environment thus rendering it safer. Every day precautions are taken to prevent accidents while travelling — for instance pedestrians and drivers comply with the rules of the road. Many of these activities are built into daily living and often are carried out without conscious effort.

Communicating

The activity of communicating not only includes the use of verbal language as in talking and writing, but also non-verbal transmission of information by facial expression and body gesture. It is also a vehicle for the transmission of emotions: long before a baby has acquired verbal language he communicates feelings such as pleasure and displeasure. Communication by touch is equally subtle although less frequently used except in intimate relationships. By its very nature, the activity of communicating permeates the whole area of interpersonal interaction and human relationships which are such an important dimension of human living.

Breathing

The very first activity of a newborn baby is breathing and the ability to do this is vital, since by this action the cells of the body will receive from the air oxygen which was previously supplied from the mother's blood. Oxygen is absolutely essential for all body cells; there is irreversible deterioration of the brain cells when they are deprived of it, even for a few minutes. Consequently, all other activities of living are entirely dependent on breathing.

Eating and drinking

A baby is born with the ability to suck and swallow so that he can obtain nourishment without which he cannot survive and grow. For most people, eating and drinking are pleasurable activities, but the fact that many people die daily from starvation even today serves as a reminder that these are activities essential to the process of living.

Eliminating

Closely associated with the ALs of eating and drinking, the activities of urinary and faecal elimination are equally essential for healthy living. In infancy, these activities occur as reflex responses to the collection of urine in the bladder and faeces in the bowel. Learning to acquire voluntary control over elimination is an important development during the early years of the life-span. Throughout the world people are socialised into eliminating in private and this contributes to many strongly held attitudes associated with this activity of living.

Personal cleansing and dressing

Cleanliness and good grooming are commended in most cultures and, apart from having pride in their appearance, people have a social responsibility to maintain personal cleanliness of body and clothing. There are a variety of activities concerned with personal cleansing; these include washing and bathing, handwashing, perineal toilet, care of hair, nails, teeth and mouth.

Controlling body temperature

The temperature of the human is maintained within a narrow range of normal. This is essential for many of the body's biological processes and it also ensures personal comfort whatever the environmental temperature. Human tissue cannot survive very long when subjected to extremes of heat or cold; trauma and even death can occur from heatstroke or hypothermia. Between these two extremes people adjust to the temperature of their environment by, for example, varying the amount of clothing and degree of activity with the objective of controlling body temperature.

Mobilising

'Mobilising' refers to the movement produced by groups of large muscles enabling people to sit, stand, walk and run. It also includes smaller movements such as those of the feet and hands and it is through the use of the smaller movements that people communicate by body gesture and facial expression. The interrelated aspects of mobilising to the other ALs should be readily apparent.

Working and playing

When not sleeping, most people are either working or playing. Play has been described as the child's work. Usually for most adults, working provides an income from which, after essential costs are met, leisure activities are financed. The activities of working and playing can have very different meanings for different individuals. The old adage 'one man's work is another man's play' illustrates this well; for example, one person might earn an income by growing flowers and vegetables to sell, whereas for another this could be a hobby. For most people to belong to work and play groups, the satisfactions from challenge and achievement, and the prevention of boredom are important aspects of working and playing.

Expressing sexuality

The specific activity which most people tend to associate with sex is sexual intercourse. Of course, this activity is an important dimension of adult relationships and essential for the propagation of the human species, but there are also many more ways in which human sexuality is expressed. Femininity and masculinity are reflected in physical appearance, strength, odour and clothes; in all forms of verbal and non-verbal communication; in family and social relationships; and in choices relating to work and play.

Sleeping

It may seem strange to consider sleeping as an 'activity' until it is realised that body processes do not stop during sleep and that sleep is essential for healthy living. All living organisms have periods of activity alternating with periods of sleep, and in human beings there is a 24-hour rhythm of sleeping and waking. Adults spend up to one-third of their lives sleeping and so, in terms of time alone, it is an important activity of living.

Dying

Because man is mortal, dying must be included amongst the activities of living. Indeed, it can be said that the process of living is a fatal one and that the final act of living is dying.

OTHER DIMENSIONS OF LIVING

Even from such a brief introduction to the various activities of living, it is clear that conceptualising living as an amalgam of activities is a helpful way of beginning to think about the complex process of living. Although the ALs are the focus of the model of living (Fig. 2.1), several other dimensions of living are included in it since they affect the ALs.

Circumstances affecting living

Not only is a person's position on the life-span relative to his position on the dependence/independence continuum for each AL, but also to his current circumstances.

Not all children are born with the capacity to become independent in all the ALs; some people are physically or mentally handicapped. However, in such circumstances, the individual is seldom totally dependent and progress can be made along the dependence/independence continuum to that person's optimum performance of each AL. And sometimes even if a person is born with the potential for complete independence, circumstances in the environment prevent or delay it. For example, poor housing conditions or lack of sensory stimulation can play a part in denying a person the

Activities of living
preventing
comforting
seeking

Maintaining a safe environment
Communicating
Breathing
Eating and drinking
Eliminating
Personal cleansing and dressing
Controlling body temperature
Mobilising
Working and playing
Expressing sexuality
Sleeping
Dying

Conception ●————— Life-span —————► Death

Totally dependent ◄————— Continuum —————► Totally independent

Fig. 2.1 Model of living

Life-span of living

Living is concerned with the whole of a person's life, his *life-span* from conception to death. The life-span is shown in the model by an arrow which indicates the direction of movement along it. As a person moves along this life-span he is continually changing and every aspect of living is influenced by physical, intellectual, emotional and social changes.

Dependence/independence in living

Because there are periods in life when a person cannot yet, or can no longer, perform certain activities of living, each individual could be said to have a *dependent/independent* continuum for each activity along which movement can take place in either direction, as shown in the model.

Newborn babies are dependent upon others for help with almost every activity of living. From this stage of almost total dependence, each child according to his capacity can be visualised as gradually moving along the continuum towards the independent pole for each AL. At five years of age the picture might look like Figure 2.2: independence has been acquired in the ALs of breathing, eliminating, controlling body temperature, mobilising and sleeping, whereas the child is far from independent in the ALs of communicating and maintaining a safe environment, for example. This idea can be applied to a person in any age group.

opportunity to develop independence in some of the ALs, such as personal cleansing and communicating.

The activities of living

The group of ALs which have already been introduced are listed on the model and, indeed, the ALs are the main focus of living used in this model. Everyone carries them out, but does so differently.

Individuality in living

Each individual develops uniquely and a person's individuality is reflected in his performance of the activities of living, influencing:

- how he carries out the AL
- how often he carries out the AL
- where he carries out the AL
- when he carries out the AL
- why he carries out the AL in a particular way
- what he knows about the AL
- what he believes about the AL.

Not only do these aspects highlight the individualised style of all ALs, but they reveal their complex nature. Yet even this does not show all the complexity because there are other dimensions which have to be considered in relation to the ALs.

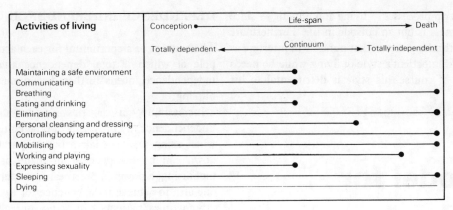

Fig. 2.2 Model of living: dependence/independence at five years old

Types of activities

In everyday life, many of the activities performed are *preventing activities*; handwashing before eating or cooking and after eliminating prevents food poisoning and the spread of infection and shows how an activity can be preventive in nature. Equally, a negative activity can be preventive; for example, refraining from smoking helps to prevent many kinds of illness all of which may lessen a person's independence in his ALs.

In the process of living, people also carry out activities which are essentially *comforting in nature*. When a person moves from his optimum level of health, as for instance when he has a severe cold, he carries out such comforting activities as keeping warm, resting in bed and taking hot drinks and nourishing meals. Physical, psychological and social comfort cannot be neglected; they are important to the health of all human beings.

Many of the activities which are carried out daily can be described as *seeking activities*. Young children are usually inveterate seekers, curious about everything in their environment and eager to find ways of mastering the many skills which must be acquired along the road to independence. Indeed, throughout the life-span individuals engage in seeking activities in their pursuit of knowledge and new experiences.

Priorities among ALs

Even from a quick consideration of what each AL involves it is clear that, although every AL is important in the process of living, some are more vital to life than others. The activity of breathing is of prime importance.

The priority which some ALs have over others is reflected in theories of human needs, for example the analysis of human needs by Abraham Maslow (1970), a well-known American psychologist. He categorised needs and then arranged the categories in order of priority creating a hierarchy of human needs. At the bottom of this are the *physiological needs*, including those for oxygen, water, food, elimination, temperature control and sleep. Next come *safety and security needs* which include things such as adequate shelter and a safe and familiar environment. *Needs for love and belonging* make up

the next category, these being human desires for human interaction, companionship and love. *Self-esteem needs* are fulfilled by frequent feed-back from others that one is valued as a person and at the top of the hierarchy are the *needs for self-actualisation* which refer to the fulfilment of one's ambitions and human potential.

The usual way of illustrating the hierarchy of human needs is by drawing a pyramid to infer the order of priority, those in the lowest category requiring to be at least minimally fulfilled before motivation is established to seek fulfilment of needs in the second category, and so on.

Occasionally, as may happen during illness, the higher needs may be submerged or engulfed by lower ones. As an example, after a serious accident, fulfilment of physiological and safety needs becomes of paramount importance and submerges all others. This example helps to establish that consideration of current priority of an individual's needs is an important part of the concept of basic human needs.

Throughout this book, however, the focus of living and nursing is not on needs but on the activities of living because they are the observable behavioural manifestations of basic human needs. People behave according to the current priority; when they are hungry they eat and drink; when they are satisfied they carry out other activities which bring pleasure and self-fulfilment. This is an example of attending to a mainly 'biological' AL before attending to those ALs which are more 'psychosocial' in nature.

Using the model of living, an account has been given of a way of conceptualising the process of living, a process which can be seen to have many dimensions. Basically man is envisaged as carrying out various activities during a life-span from conception to death. His main objective is to attain self-fulfilment and maximum independence in each activity of living within the limitations set by his particular circumstances. He also carries out many activities of a preventing, comforting and seeking nature and he appropriately alters priorities among the activities of living. In these ways, the individual endeavours to be healthy and independent in the process of living.

This way of thinking about living will now be transferred to nursing. It is highly desirable to develop a similar way of thinking about the two processes — living and nursing — since for most people, illness is but an episode in life. Furthermore this similar way of thinking means that nurses will interfere as little as possible with a patient's style of living while he needs nursing — unless, of course, his style is detrimental to his health!

The model for nursing

Inasmuch as there are preventing, comforting and seeking activities interrelated with the ALs in the model of living, there are preventing, comforting and dependent components interrelated with the AL component of nursing in the model for nursing (Fig. 2.3). The links between these two models are explained in the following discussion.

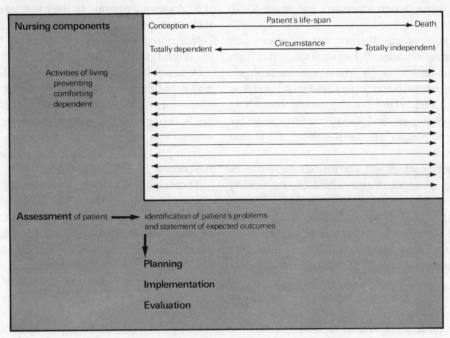

Fig. 2.3 A model for nursing

PATIENT'S LIFE-SPAN

The patient's life-span is represented on the model; it is a reminder that nursing is concerned with people of all ages and that an individual may come into contact with nursing services at any stage of his life-span. Some nursing services are specifically concerned with one particular stage of the life-span; midwifery is the term used to describe nursing related to pregnancy and childbirth, paediatric nursing concentrates on nursing children, and geriatric nursing specialises in nursing elderly people.

DEPENDENCE/INDEPENDENCE OF PATIENTS

The concept of a continuum for each activity of living, at one pole of which is total dependence and at the other, total independence, needs further development when considering nursing.

Increasingly, it is possible to maintain a person's 'independence' by providing special equipment. For example, when using a wheelchair a person paralysed from the waist down can be independent in many aspects of the AL of mobilising; a powered prosthesis may permit a child with only one arm to achieve independence for eating and drinking.

Sometimes patients can strive unrealistically to maintain their independence in certain activities of living and need to be encouraged, maybe only temporarily, to accept a dependent role. The fierce independence of the older person is occasionally not in his best interest; the same is true of the acutely ill patient.

A very important aspect of nursing is assessing a patient's level of independence in all activities of living and judging in which direction, and by what amount, he should be assisted to move along his dependent/independent continua and what help he requires to meet the objectives set.

CIRCUMSTANCES AFFECTING PATIENTS

Some of the circumstances which can prevent movement towards maximum independence, and some which can produce movement towards dependence even though independence had been achieved, were mentioned in the discussion of this aspect of the model of living. There are some additional circumstances which need consideration for nursing. The relevant items are:

● physical, psychological and social environment
● disability and disturbed physiology, both of which can be congenital or acquired, resulting in either predominantly physical or predominantly mental dysfunction
● tissue changes which can be pathological or degenerative
● accident
● infection.

COMPONENTS OF NURSING

Nursing is particularly concerned with patient's activities of living. The 'AL component' of nursing incorporates in many instances the 'preventing', 'comforting' and 'dependent' components. Each will be discussed separately, but in reality they are so closely interrelated that elements from each component can be present in any single nursing activity.

The AL component of nursing
The AL component of nursing includes all those nursing activities which are carried out in relation to the patient's activities of living.

The objectives of these nursing activities are in most instances to preserve as far as possible the patient's usual habits and routines associated with each AL. Personal habits and attitudes are often deeply entrenched and having to make changes during an episode of illness or hospitalisation can be a source of stress and anxiety. Nursing activities aim to minimise this possibility.

However, in some instances the patient's established habits relating to an AL may have contributed to his health problem or could do so in the future. An excellent example of this is overeating which may result in obesity and contributes to many physical and mental disorders. In this case, nursing activities for the AL of eating and drinking would be aimed at changing the patient's attitude and habits to result in the measurable desirable outcome, loss of weight.

In general, the AL component of nursing is concerned with helping patients with particular problems related to activities of living. The problems may be the result of a change of environment and routine, or difficulty in achieving or maintaining independence, or changes in usual habit or mode of carrying out the AL, or discomforts associated with the AL. The nursing activities involved may range from simply providing some helpful information or equipment to actually carrying out certain tasks of everyday living for the patient. A range of patients' problems and related nursing activities associated with each activity of living are identified and discussed in Section 3 of *The Elements of Nursing*.

The preventing component of nursing
One of Florence Nightingale's well-known statements is 'the hospital shall do the patient no harm'. There are many potential sources of harm in hospitals and its prevention should be a part of every nursing activity. Undue stress and anxiety can be harmful and delay recovery; a hospital-acquired infection produces a secondary problem which may hamper recovery from the illness which precipitated the patient's admission to hospital. Confinement to bed is fraught with possible complications; these are potential problems and their prevention is an essential part of nursing.

Many patients on leaving hospital require to have the knowledge which can help to prevent the recurrence of the treated condition so teaching patients about prevention is an important nursing responsibility. The emphasis in health education is primarily on promoting health but the corollary is prevention of ill-health: all nurses should be health educators.

The comforting component of nursing
This component includes what many people associate with nursing and think of as the 'art' of nursing. Simple activities such as helping a patient into a comfortable position, taking time over the patient's personal appearance, putting a meal tray in the most accessible place for the patient to take his food, ensuring that his locker is within easy reach of his preferred hand or remembering to pass on a message of greeting from a relative who phoned are examples of comforting activities. The objective of all activities in this component of nursing is to achieve the patient's maximum physical comfort and enhance his ability to cope, physically and mentally, with his indisposition.

The dependent component of nursing
This component is derived from the 'seeking' activities in the model of living on the premise that when a person is ill he *seeks medical help and may consequently require nursing*. The tasks in this component are the dependent part of the nurse's role and are considered by some people to contribute to the 'technical' part of her role.

The administration of drugs is an example of an activity in the dependent component of nursing. The doctor prescribes medications, specifying the dose, time and route of administration. By custom in hospital the nurse administers the medications, strictly adhering to the doctor's prescription. However, some drugs are prescribed to be given 'when necessary' and this involves skilful judgment on the part of the nurse. Often nurses help patients to learn to administer their own medications, usually at home; the medications may have to be taken orally, inhaled or injected.

Many treatments such as surgical dressings are prescribed by the doctor to be carried out by the nurse. Yet other treatments, such as passive exercise of particular muscles or limbs are performed by physiotherapists and other members of the multiprofessional team. Sometimes the nurse must also assist with these treatments, perhaps supervising or helping the patient with exercises in the absence of the physiotherapist.

Most tests are medically prescribed. For example, testing urine is carried out by the nurse at the doctor's request. Sometimes the nurse assists the doctor with tests, such as lumbar puncture, by preparing the equipment, explaining the procedure to the patient, and looking after his physical and mental comfort before, during and after the test.

Even in this dependent component of nursing, the nurse is concerned with comforting and preventing activities as they interrelate with the activities of living.

THE PROCESS OF NURSING

The model for nursing is helpful in identifying and grouping nursing activities and in showing how closely nursing is associated with the process of living. In the application to practice of this theoretical model, it is clear that several steps are involved when nursing activities are carried out. First, the patient must be assessed; nursing intervention must be planned; the plan must be implemented; and, in order to maintain effectiveness and continually re-think the plan, evaluation must be carried out.

The process is not new in nursing; the 'good nurse' has always used it. Often, however, she did not analyse what she was doing, nor did she verbalise the phases of the process as she carried out each nursing activity, so some learners found it difficult to appreciate the rapidly executed cognitive aspects of the task observed. Learners were often unaware that the experienced nurse had selected out of several possible alternatives, one particular regime for a particular patient, and were therefore unable to comprehend the reason.

Also nurses did not commit to paper their rapid thinking about assessing, planning, implementing and evaluating. If all nurses begin to document and retain nursing data, it will not only be useful for nursing subsequent patients, but it will provide evidence of:

- nursing's body of knowledge
- the value and prestige of the nurse-initiated components of nursing
- the evaluated effectiveness of specific nursing interventions
- the decision-making aspects underlying nursing activities, a criterion used by managers when assessing status and earnings.

Assessment
Activities of living (ALs) can be used as the criteria for which assessment data are collected. Data about the patient's ALs need not be collected in any particular order and in some circumstances not all ALs need to be considered. It is often inadvisable to collect very detailed information at the first encounter with a patient; indeed it is likely that further

pertinent information will be forthcoming at each interaction with the patient as increasing rapport is established. Of course, in life-threatening emergency situations, only minimal essential data are collected before the patient is transferred to the operating theatre or before life-saving measures are implemented.

Whatever type of admission form, assessment form, nursing history or nursing Kardex is used for recording purposes, the nurse needs to be very sensitive about where, when and how she collects information from patients. Part of the skill of nursing is recognising when, and knowing how to collect information.

Some patients may not want to divulge information about certain aspects of their daily living, wishing to retain as much privacy as possible. The nurse can explain that certain information is essential if the necessary treatment is to be provided and that other information may be relevant in identifying potential, as well as actual, health problems. Nurses who have used nursing assessments usually experience favourable patients' reactions to the opportunity of giving information and talking with a nurse.

However, it may also be important to reassure patients that information given to nurses is regarded as confidential. Confidentiality is often a loosely used word these days; rather than using this term, it may be advisable to state exactly where information will be stored and who has access to it, reassuring the patient that information is confined to the health care team.

Some hospitals are experimenting with patient-completed assessment forms. Aspinall (1975) carried out a comparative study and found that the data thus obtained compared favourably with information collected from the nursing interview. But obviously not all patients would be able or willing to participate in such an exercise.

To help readers to develop skills in assessing, a broad view will be given of the sort of information relevant to consider in a nursing assessment. Examples are given of the type of questions that the nurse in her role of assessor might bear in mind when interacting with a patient. The patient need not be asked all the questions; in fact the nurse will obtain many 'answers' by astute observation — some of which of course will need to be confirmed by the patient. The list of questions is not exhaustive and many others will be seen to be appropriate as the nurse becomes more skilled at assessing patients. The objectives in collecting data about patients' ALs are to discover:

- previous routines
- what the patient can do for himself
- what the patient cannot do for himself
- problems (actual/potential) and previous coping mechanisms.

Assessing ability to maintain a safe environment is of particular importance if the patient has any sensory impairment: poor vision, poor hearing, inability to smell, or loss of peripheral sensation. How does the blind person prevent injury? What precautions does the deaf person take to avoid accident? Has the patient who cannot smell developed any compensatory activities, or taken any precautions, to make his environment safe? What activities does the paraplegic patient carry out to prevent pressure sores? Whether they are in hospital or at home, what can physically and/or mentally handicapped patients do to keep their environment safe? Assessing ability to maintain a safe environment is an important function of the community nurses, especially those visiting children or elderly people. Is the floor trip-free? Are the hygiene standards sufficient to prevent infection? Are fires guarded? Are medicines, poisons and sharp instruments stored safely?

Assessing communicating skills can take place at every interaction between nurse and patient. It has to be remembered that communicating is one of the ALs which is very much affected by such factors as stage of development, level of intelligence, personality traits and current mood. The following examples are general questions which will apply to most adults. Can he see and hear adequately? If not, is there dysfunction of right or left eye/ear or both? What factors does he find helpful/unhelpful when people are talking with him? Does he use any corrective aids? Are they in good working order? Is his speech audible, coherent, fluent, confident, inaudible, incoherent, interrupted in its flow, nervous? Does he appear to have a limited/average/extensive vocabulary? Can he read and write? Does he appear to be comfortable/uncomfortable with eye contact? Does he gesticulate excessively/acceptably/sparingly? Is he gregarious by nature or more fond of his own company?

Assessing a patient's breathing may involve simply ensuring that breathing has not stopped or, more usually for various reasons, counting and recording the number of respirations per minute. Given that the patient is breathing, the nurse needs to discover: does he have any difficulty with breathing? Does he have any pain or discomforts associated with breathing? Can he describe the pain? When does it occur? What increases/decreases the pain? For other patients the nurse will need to ask: does he cough? If so, when? Does coughing produce sputum? Can he describe the sputum? What increases/decreases the coughing? Does the atmosphere at work exacerbate the coughing? Is his breathing ever 'wheezy'? Does he get colds often/sometimes/seldom/never? Does he smoke? If so, does he smoke cigarettes, cigars, a pipe? How many cigarettes, cigars, or how much tobacco? Does he smoke daily? What factors increase/decrease his usual smoking habits? At what age did he start smoking? Has he ever given it up? If so, for how long? What made him start again? What does he know about the ill effects of smoking?

Assessing eating and drinking routines is a necessary part of an admission assessment so that related nursing can be planned appropriately. What is the person's usual diet, dietary likes and dislikes? Are any dietary modifications observed? If so, are these medical, religious, sociocultural or personal-choice modifications? Is he able to eat and drink independently? Are any aids needed to maintain independence? If the patient is a child, exact details of his dependence/independence will be necessary. Does the patient have any problems or discomforts associated with eating and drinking? If so, can he describe them, their relationship to food/fluid intake, and what relieves them? Is he overnourished/well nourished/undernourished? Is his weight in keeping with his height, build and age? What are his usual eating and drinking routines: does he eat alone or with others; where does he usually eat and drink? Because most people enjoy talking about this AL, information about it is usually relatively easy to obtain.

Assessing a patient's eliminating habits is a necessary nursing function even though his current health problem is not associated with bowel or urinary dysfunction. But there may well be a long-term problem with constipation or recurrent cystitis and this may be elicited from the assessment. Many people find it embarrassing to talk about elimination and the nurse needs to broach the topic with sensitivity and phrase the questions carefully to avoid embarrassment. The nurse can help the patient by saying that different people use different words (water, urine, voiding; stool, faeces, bowel movement, bowels open) and using the ones with which the patient is familiar. At what time does he pass urine? What factors increase/decrease this frequency? Can he estimate how much he passes each time? What factors increase/decrease this amount? Does he have any difficulty in passing urine? Can he describe it? What increases/decreases the difficulty? Can he describe the urine? What is his normal bowel habit? What factors increase/decrease this frequency? Can he describe the faeces? Does he have any problems or discomforts associated with defaecation? From patients who excrete via a stoma, the nurse will discover how they cope at home, and whether or not they will continue to cope independently in hospital.

Assessing personal cleansing and dressing is possible by observing the results of these activities; ill-cared-for clothes may be an indication of financial hardship or a lack of self-esteem which can characterise exhaustion or mental illness. Shabby but clean clothes may be an indication of financial hardship. Clothes inappropriate for the climatic conditions may be indicative of inability to appreciate or respond appropriately to changes in the temperature of the external environment. It may be tactful to preface questions about personal hygiene by a remark such as 'What do we need to know so that we interfere as little as possible with your usual hygiene habits?' As with all the ALs, the nurse needs to be sensitive and skilful at recognising a patient's discomfort; some people are embarrassed at revealing that their home does not have a bathroom, while others are proud to proclaim that all the family have kept themselves clean without a bathroom. The objective in nurses collecting information about patients' personal cleansing activities is to permit such usual routines as bathing, handwashing, hairwashing and mouth cleaning to continue — unless a routine is found to be prejudicial to health. In this instance, instruction may be necessary so the nursing plan should include appropriate aspects of health education.

Assessing control of body temperature is not as amenable to questioning as many of the other ALs, but data can be obtained by observation and measurement. Observation may reveal flushing of the skin, excessive perspiration, the presence of goose flesh, shivering, and excessively hot or cold hands and/or feet. If an accurate assessment of body temperature is required, this may be measured with a clinical thermometer.

When assessing mobilising, initially it is necessary to observe whether or not there are any apparent musculoskeletal abnormalities. But people vary enormously in their exercise habits related to home, work and play activities so it is important to broach these various aspects of mobilising with the patient. Lack of exercise can contribute to some kinds of health problems and again inclusion of remedial health education in the nursing plan may be relevant. The patient who has an obvious mobilising problem may have a walking aid or wheelchair, and this will make it easier to discuss how he copes and what help he needs. Questions can be asked about impaired movement and pain. For example, is there any stiffness of the joints? If so, which ones? Does he know what causes it? Does he have any muscular pain or discomfort? If so, where? What increases/decreases it? Does he have any joint pains? If so, which joints? What increases/decreases the pain?

Assessing working and playing routines is necessary because they may well have implications for nursing. What is the patient's occupation? Where does he work? Can he describe the working conditions? By the way he responds the nurse may well discover whether he finds work challenging or boring and she would recognise whether or not the working conditions might have contributed to his accident or illness. There may be cues indicating difficulty in work or social relationships because of personality problems and these may have contributed to the illness. How far from home is his work and by which means does he travel? How many hours does he work? Does he work overtime and if so, how much? How much time does he devote to playing activities? What are his hobbies? When did he last have a holiday from work? Will he be bored while off sick? Obtaining details of play activities is essential if the patient is a child: what stage of development has he reached? What are his favourite toys and books?

Assessment of the AL of expressing sexuality will require a different approach, according to circumstances. In a gynaecological or genito-urinary unit, it may be important for the nurse to obtain information about sexual function, and the effects of the patient's health problem on his/her sexual feelings. It is likely that a female patient admitted to hospital for treatment of a gynaecological complaint will expect to be asked, and be prepared to answer, fairly direct questions about her menstrual cycle, contraceptive practice, parity and pregnancies. In contrast, such questions, understandably, might alarm and embarrass a patient admitted for treatment of varicose veins, for example! However, now that it is beginning to be understood that many different sorts of health problems

may affect sexual function or feelings of sexuality, it is essential for nurses to be able to obtain relevant data which will help them to identify patients' problems and anxieties concerning this AL, if it is appropriate to do so.

Assessing sleeping routines at an early stage is important so that nurses have information on which to base nursing activities aimed at promoting sleep. Patients are not usually admitted to hospital because of a sleep problem as such, but adequate sleep is important for progress towards recovery, whatever the reason for admission. What is the patient's pre-sleep routine? At what time does he retire to bed? At what time does he usually go to sleep? Does he waken during the sleep period; if so, at what time does he waken? What does he do to get to sleep again? Does he consider himself a good/average/poor sleeper? Does he feel refreshed/unrefreshed on waking? What is his usual 'morning mood'? Does he have to adjust his sleep to shift work? Does he take sleeping pills: always/sometimes/seldom/never? If so, does he know which ones? Does he have them with him? What factors increase/decrease his sleep?

Assessing the needs of the dying and the dying person's relatives is a very important role of the nurse in hospital and in the community. Constant sensitivity and astute observation are necessary to recognise whether or not the patient/relative wants to talk about the many anxieties associated with death, dying and bereavement. Assessment of the specific nursing needs of the dying patient may be carried out in relation to each AL separately, as previously discussed.

Assessment, then, is not a once-only activity, or a rigid routine carried out at a particular time. It is a continuous or ongoing activity as nurses are constantly observing and interacting with patients. The main purpose of a nursing assessment is identification of the patients' actual or potential problems that are amenable to nursing help. Apart from the problems obvious to the patient, there can be a nurse-perceived problem of which the patient is unaware: for example, infestation with head lice. It must be noted so that it can be treated, otherwise lice may be transmitted to others. In other instances, the patient may wish to decide whether or not the problem, previously not apparent to him, should be treated.

The data from assessment are analysed and the patients' problems, both actual and potential should be clearly stated. For each actual/potential problem a goal or patient outcome is then decided. Discussion with the patient whenever it is possible, and perhaps with his family, may help in stating feasible patient outcomes that can be anticipated. Patient outcomes are the goals or objectives of nursing intervention. They should be stated in observable and/or measurable terms so that they can be used as criteria in the 'evaluation phase' of nursing.

To give some examples, if a patient's problem is constipation, the patient outcome would be a return to the usual bowel habit in which stools are not difficult or painful to pass. If the problem is incontinence of urine, the desirable patient outcome would be continence of urine. A potential problem for any patient whose mobility is severely restricted, whether he is in bed or in a chair, is the development of a deep vein thrombosis in the lower limb, the presence of which causes pain and inflammation. The patient outcome stated in observable terms would be unswollen, pain-free lower limbs at the same temperature as the rest of the skin.

Planning

A clear statement of the expected outcomes leads naturally into the second phase of the process, planning for nursing intervention to achieve the expected patient outcomes. Planning includes consideration of:

- available resources, such as:
  physical environment
  equipment
  personnel
- possible alternative nursing interventions.

When planning for the most appropriate *physical environment*, a decision may have to be made as to whether the person would be best nursed at home or in hospital. Should the patient have an infection and have to be barrier-nursed, a single room would be preferable to a shared one. Planning also includes details of such factors as the distance between the bed and the toilet if the patient has to make frequent visits.

Availability of suitable *equipment* can have an important effect on planning nursing. Variable height beds may help to prevent accidents to frail and disabled patients. Aids to mobilising, such as walking frames and wheelchairs, may be necessary. Special utensils have to be considered when patients have certain physical problems with feeding.

Consideration of *available personnel* will include not only numbers of nursing staff but also their level of preparation and their previous nursing experience. This has to be related to the planned nursing activities and especially to the nursing workload. In the inevitable instances of shortage of nursing staff on a particular work shift, existing personnel must decide which nursing activities can safely be omitted for that shift. It is safer to do essential nursing activities well than to attempt all desirable activities and risk not only sub-standard nursing but a lowering of the nurses' morale due to lack of job satisfaction. When patients are nursed at home, or their transfer home from hospital is imminent, the availability of family and neighbours should be considered as a resource.

When patients are nursed at home information about available support services is needed. Such resources as home-helps, volunteer workers, night nursing staff, laundry services and meals-on-wheels may have to be considered.

Possible alternative nursing interventions may be determined by the availability of resources. Decisions have to be made about such things as, for example, should the patient use a commode at the bedside independently or walk 15 steps to the toilet assisted by two nurses? Walking would perhaps best meet the patient's mobility needs but it involves two nurses at the required times. Choice of intervention may also be made on the basis of evidence of best known effectiveness: for example, regular relief of pressure is known to be preferable to an alternative commonly in use — 'pressure care rounds'.

Having considered the resources, the next procedure is to make decisions about what the nurse and (when possible) the patient agree to do to achieve the expected outcomes related to each of the patient's problems. For those activities which the patient agrees to do, the associated nursing activity is supervision. A *nursing plan* is then made of all the necessary nursing activities stated in sufficient detail so that any other nurse, on reading the plan, would be aware of and carry out the planned nursing activities. There is no argument against this being essential since no one nurse can be on duty throughout the 24 hours and sufficient detail of the plans made for each patient cannot possibly be conveyed in verbal reports.

A nursing plan is not a static thing but requires continual revision as additional data are collected from ongoing assessment. Also, when evaluation reveals that an expected outcome has not been achieved for a particular patient's problem, there may well have to be a change in the nursing activities and this must be recorded in the nursing plan.

Social changes which have affected the nursing profession, such as decreased working hours, and an increase in both annual leave and the use of part-time staff, have made it essential for nurses to develop the skill of communicating by writing adequate nursing plans. If such trends continue, it may well be that the nursing plan will assume even greater importance as a means of communication between nurses. And furthermore, assessing a patient and writing a nursing plan help the nurse and patient to know each other. This, in turn, aids the establishment of a satisfactory nurse/patient relationship, the unique basis of the nursing contribution to a patient's health care.

Implementation

The third phase of the process of nursing is actually carrying out the prepared plan. A day-to-day record must be made of the nursing activities implemented: when they were carried out, and by whom, together with any relevant information e.g., the patient may have experienced nausea soon after administration of the analgesic drug prescribed for him. An 'implementation sheet', 'flow chart' or 'record sheet' can be used for the purpose of recording the nursing activities implemented. Whatever the format, it is important for nurses to consider this recording as a data-collecting exercise. The data must be retained as they will become nursing's data bank on which retrospective research can be carried out to fill many of the gaps in our knowledge of nursing.

Evaluation

It is difficult to justify the existence of nursing if it cannot be demonstrated that it benefits the recipient in specific ways, hence the fourth phase in the process of nursing, evaluation. The expected patient outcomes, already stated, are the criteria used in evaluation; without them, evaluation is a misnomer. Some nurses are confused about assessing and evaluating; some of the skills used are common to both activities, but evaluating involves comparison against an objective — the stated patient outcome. When the expected outcomes are not achieved, there has to be reassessment of that problem with the patient.

At the Congress in Tokyo in 1977, the president of the International Council of Nurses chose the watchword *accountability* for nurses for the next quadrennium. The two crucial issues in nursing accountability are: statement of expected patient outcomes and evaluation of whether or not they have been achieved. They are crucial because the evaluative component of nursing cannot take place unless preceded by a statement of expectation. By using the process of nursing, nurses should be able to render accountability for the service which they provide.

PATIENT ASSESSMENT FORM

The Patient Assessment Form used throughout this book has as its rationale, recording of the patient's biographical and health data on the left-hand side and data about the patient's ALs on the right-hand side (Fig. 2.4, pp 16-17). As will be shown in the nine patient studies, these two sets of data do have relevance to each other. Use of each side of the form will be discussed separately.

Biographical and health data

As there may be two patients with the same *surname* it is necessary to write out the *forenames* in long hand and to avoid using initials for any of them. It is customary in some hospitals to ask the patient what form of address he would prefer the staff to use because being addressed in the usual way can help a patient to retain his sense of personal identity and dignity.

All cities have their affluent and disadvantaged areas so an *address* can alert the staff to possible problems which the patient might have on discharge, with ALs such as mobilising or maintaining a safe environment. An address may give an indication of status and income which could be relevant to the nursing plan, e.g., a patient in the low income group who requires an expensive high protein diet.

Likewise the *type of accommodation* could well have relevance to the nursing plan; if a chronically breathless patient lives in a fourth floor flat that does not have a lift, arrangement of an early appointment with the medical social worker will be a necessary nursing activity. When patients are on diuretic drugs the type of toilet accommodation is obviously relevant.

Information about *family/others* who live at the patient's address may reveal that he lives alone, a factor which could influence the planning of his rehabilitation and the date of his discharge. It could also inform the staff of his anxiety and fear about the house being unoccupied, or especially in the winter

months about problems such as burst water pipes. In other instances, should a telephone call have to be made by a nurse to this address, it is important for her to know to whom she might be speaking.

The name of the *next of kin*, is, of course, essential information; even the knowledge that there is no next of kin is important and relevant. It is possible that a patient separated from his wife may not want her to be contacted without his permission and this would be noted.

Information about the *significant others* in a patient's life can have relevance to planning the patient's nursing. Knowledge about 'relatives/dependents' may result in such items as 'Talk with patient about handicapped daughter' being written on the nursing plan. Information about 'helpers' may be useful when planning the patient's discharge. And a note about 'visitors' will alert members of nursing staff to help a patient, who is likely to have many visitors, to plan a visiting rota. In the instance of a patient having no one to visit him, the nurse might offer a volunteer visitor. The term 'significant others' is sufficiently broad, so that it can include all possible relationships.

The patient's *occupation* may not only affect the planning of a rehabilitation programme for him but also alert the nurse to think about how for instance a low income might be affecting his family, and she could offer to make an appointment with the medical social worker. On the other hand, the occupation could be a contributory factor to the reason for admission, e.g., dust from coal mining being a precursor to chronic respiratory disease.

It is important for nurses to know of any *religious beliefs and practices* which have implications for the nursing plan. The patient may or may not wish to attend the services in the hospital chapel, or participate in a ward communion service, or be visited by a particular hospital chaplain or his own minister of religion. But religious beliefs can have direct bearing on the ALs of eating and drinking, personal cleansing and dressing.

Collection of *health data* can be carried out prior to the assessment interview, indeed they and many of the biographical data can be collected from the patient's case notes which usually results in a more relaxed interview. Information about the patient's health data permits the nurse to gain understanding of his knowledge about, and his attitude to, his health status. It is important for nurses to know his perception of his current health status e.g., his understanding of the nature of a chronic disorder. It is useful for nurses to know his understanding of the reason for his admission, for instance whether or not he knows that he has been scheduled for an investigation under general anaesthetic and not an operation. He may or may not know his medical diagnosis and past medical history, and in any case these should be checked with the medical notes.

Allergies are an important consideration. There are so many things (adhesive bandages, particular foods, pollens, feathers and drugs) to which people are allergic and it is important to record these.

It is useful to know whether the patient has undergone recently any *significant life crisis* such as starting new employment, changing house or school, marriage, divorce or bereavement; it is known that such crises can affect health adversely.

The biographical and health data, collected as described, in addition to providing essential information about the patient, will suggest topics obviously requiring further exploration in the more detailed assessment of each AL.

Activities of living data
On the right-hand side of the Patient Assessment Form, data about each of the patient's ALs are recorded. Earlier in this section we gave examples of the sort of questions to bear in mind at the assessment interview and indeed at all times, since it cannot be too strongly stressed that assessment is an ongoing process. The objective is to discover the patient's previous routines, what he can and cannot do for himself in relation to each AL. After analysis of the data the patient's problems are identified and written on the right-hand side of the form. Potential problems are identified by the sign (p).

The Patient Assessment Form was used in each of the nine studies which follow.

REFERENCES

Aspinall M J 1975 Development of a patient-completed questionnaire and its comparison with the nursing interview. Nursing Research 24(5): 377–381
Maslow A H 1970 Motivation and personality, 2nd edn. Harper and Row, New York
Roper N 1976 Clinical experience in nurse education. Churchill Livingstone, Edinburgh

Figure 2.4 is on pages 16–17.

Patient Assessment Form

Date of admission   Date of assessment

Surname   Forenames

Male ☐   Age ☐   Single/Married/Widowed   Prefers to be addressed as

Female ☐   Date of birth   Other

Address of usual residence

Type of accommodation

Family/Others at this residence

Next of kin   Name   Address

                     Relationship   Tel. no.

Significant others   Relatives/Dependents

                     Helpers

                     Visitors

Occupation

Religious beliefs and relevant practices

Patient's perception of current health status

Reason for admission/referral

Medical diagnosis

Past medical history

Allergies   Significant life crises

Fig. 2.4 Patient Assessment Form

Assessment of Activities of Living

Date

AL	Usual routines: what he/she can and cannot do independently	Patient's problems (actual/potential) (p) = potential
● Maintaining a safe environment		
● Communicating		
● Breathing		
● Eating and drinking		
● Eliminating		
● Personal cleansing and dressing		
● Controliing body temperature		
● Mobilising		
● Working and playing		
● Expressing sexuality		
● Sleeping		
● Dying		

3
A study of a diabetic patient
using the model for nursing

Annina B. Mayhew and Elizabeth Y. Howie

All the great revolutions in men's lives are made in thought. When a change takes place in men's thought, action follows the direction of thought as a ship follows the direction given by its rudder.

Tolstoy

The authors

THE NURSE TEACHER

For some ten months I had been attempting to use the activities of living in my teaching because this framework supported the idea that among other things the nurse assists the individual patient in the performance of those activities contributing to health which he would normally perform for himself. This means that the nurse must be aware of the patient's normal pattern of behaviour before she can identify the problems. This also allows her to assess the need for health education and once aware of that need, it can be included in planned nursing activities. So I had been thinking in terms of the Roper, Logan and Tierney model for ten months and had just begun to introduce the first year students to nursing using this approach. It had been a major exercise to re-think the presentation of the content in the entire first year programme but it was rewarding. The new students were responding very positively to the use of the activities of living as a framework on which to build their nursing knowledge and skills, and could quickly see the relevance of discussing communicating, eating and drinking, mobilising, sleeping and so on — activities with which they themselves were familiar, and indeed almost took for granted. Till then, they had scarcely stopped to consider the many factors involved.

I had also been studying and writing about the process of nursing over a period of a few years, and considering how this systematic way of thinking about nursing, and organising nursing activities could be used by student nurses. So it had not been too difficult for me to consider the nursing process mode of thinking within an activities of living model when devising the first-year programme.

Unfortunately it is still widely held that a great divide exists between what is taught in college and what is practised in the clinical area and as a teacher, this has caused me great concern. Since the importance of knowledge lies in its use, I had to encourage student nurses to use their knowledge for the benefit of the patient. It seemed to me that if the activities of living framework and the process of nursing were used in the college and in the clinical areas, it would focus on how theory can be translated into practice and it would highlight the nursing contribution to patient care.

I, therefore, welcomed the opportunity to work on this study with a colleague in a clinical area. It gave me the opportunity to work with actual patients and not just in a theoretical setting and would, I hoped, help me in my teaching.

THE SISTER, DIABETIC UNIT

On being asked to practise the ideas presented in *The Elements of Nursing,* I had at first to familiarise myself with the book and its approach as I did not have any experience of using the process of nursing or the model. This took quite a long time. I was very impressed by the approach in the book and felt that there definitely was a need to improve our nursing practice and also the way in which it was recorded. I liked the idea of approaching nursing from an assessment of the patient's total needs rather than starting from his medical condition; and I was very willing to try the 'activities of living' model to see how it would work in practice.

My responsibility within the Diabetic Unit is for the education and support of the diabetic patient and his family and to do this, I keep a checklist of relevant topics for discussion. As I am the only member of nursing staff principally concerned with education, I work closely with the dietitian and have frequent contact with the ward nursing and medical staff. Until now, however, any recording of patient education has been entered in the medical case records, and most of my communication with nursing and medical staff has been by word of mouth.

My office/clinic is adjacent to a medical ward and I have responsibility for any diabetic patient within the hospital and for all diabetic outpatients. At 11 a.m. and 4 p.m. each day, Monday to Friday, any patient wishing to attend for consultation without appointment can do so and telephone calls to me for advice and information can be accepted at any time. The policy is to admit all newly diagnosed, juvenile-onset diabetic patients to a medical ward for approximately five to ten days for stabilisation and education although the length of time varies according to the patient's physical condition and how quickly he learns about his diabetic condition. I am notified of each new admission and visit as soon as possible to get to know the patient and help him begin to understand a little about his condition. Because of the ward's proximity, it is possible to visit him at regular intervals for education and to see his relatives as often as necessary at mutually suitable times to help them adjust and learn about diabetes. In addition it is possible, personally, to follow up the patient after discharge from hospital.

It will be noted in this study that the patient was taught glucose monitoring instead of urine testing for assessment of diabetic control as this is the policy of the unit for young diabetic patients.

Introduction to the patient

Tommy, a 15-year-old boy, had felt unwell at school. He had also been very tired, wanted to keep on drinking lemonade and knew his sleep was being disturbed by having to go to the toilet on numerous occasions throughout the night. He himself told his mother he wanted to visit their doctor and when the general practitioner made the diagnosis, Tommy was referred to the Diabetic Clinic. Admission to hospital offered a 'safe' place for Tommy while his condition was brought under control and it took him away from his family until both came to terms with diabetes and its implications, and got to know something about the adjustments Tommy would be advised to make in his everyday activities.

He had a general medical examination including a number of routine investigations — chest X-ray; full blood count; ESR; ECG; viral studies; urea and electrolytes; liver function tests — and all results were within normal limits.

The biochemistry technician performed glucose profiles on the 1st, 2nd, 5th and 6th days of Tommy's sojourn and this involved taking capillary blood samples before breakfast, lunch, tea and supper. As there was no indication of ketosis on the day of admission subcutaneous injections of insulin were prescribed and, other than Mixtard insulin before breakfast and before the evening meal each day, Tommy had no medication. The actual dosage of insulin was altered by the doctor according to the glucose profile results and the injections were supervised by me. The nursing staff in the ward supervised Tommy's injections at the weekend (his 3rd and 4th day in the ward) and also performed routine urinalysis throughout his stay.

Tommy was free to wear his own outdoor clothes, and to go out of the ward for walks during his stay in hospital. Only one incident arose when Tommy ate two bars of diabetic chocolate given to him by a visitor on the Saturday; the Sorbitol content caused him to have diarrhoea. He had actually been warned of such a consequence but it seemed he had to learn his lesson the hard way.

Quite soon after admission to the diabetic ward, Tommy was asked if he would be willing to have his care described in a nursing text and he and his mother were very happy to give their permission.

Discussion on presentation of documentation

The framework of this nursing study was the result of much deliberation. The following paragraphs discuss each part of the study explaining why it has been laid out as seen in Figures 3.1—3.6, pages 22—31.

PATIENT ASSESSMENT FORM: BIOGRAPHICAL AND HEALTH DATA

The biographical data were recorded on the left-hand side of the Roper, Logan and Tierney Patient Assessment Form (PAF) and was considered adequate (Fig. 3.1, p. 22). The inclusion of the patient's perception of his own health status (which was not normally recorded) meant that the patient's point of view was immediately identifiable and this was therefore thought to be an advantage.

PATIENT ASSESSMENT FORM: ASSESSMENT OF ALs

On first using the right-hand side of the PAF, (Fig. 3.2, p. 24) thought had to be given as to what should be included in the different categories. One of the concerns was whether all the observations that one would want to make could be fitted into the headings given. In fact, in practice, this turned out to be relatively easy to overcome by referring to the guidelines in *The Elements of Nursing*.

Having assessed the patient's activities of living (first assessment), and appreciating the implications of his condition, the identification of the problems and potential problems was a natural progression, for example, Tommy said he had a great liking for sweets and had been drinking lots of lemonade, so it was obvious that having to limit his intake of sweets could be a problem.

THE GOALS

The next stage was the layout of the nursing plan to cover goals, evaluation and intervention. Because the régime he would have to follow would be lifelong, it seemed appropriate to divide the goals into short- and long-term (Fig. 3.3, p. 26). This allowed for evaluation of the patient's progress after his initial instruction in diabetic care, while acknowledging that his learning would continue at home. The evaluation of whether he had reached the short-term goal in fact was timed to assess his readiness for home. It was obvious that, once at home, he would require reinforcement and support on a regular basis until he gained confidence in coping with his condition. The long-term goals, therefore, drew attention to the need for ongoing education and allowed for re-evaluation at regular intervals. As new problems arose, other goals could be set; as problems were solved, the relevant goals could be changed or omitted. It will be noted that we did not need to set goals for the twelve ALs at this point; only six were relevant to Tommy. So we did not require a proforma. A blank sheet of paper with appropriate headings was all that was needed.

THE EVALUATION

For the evaluation column within the plan, it seemed appropriate to state the date on which the nurse could assess whether or not each short-term goal had been achieved. On that date a further complete assessment was performed (second assessment). This is the reason why the evaluation column comes before, instead of after, intervention. There were two advantages in this: firstly, the ease with which outstanding problems were noted; secondly, all twelve of the activities of living were reviewed including those which had previously been problem-free to ensure that this was still the case. The third assessment was carried out two weeks after discharge to assess progress at home. This nursing study was then terminated although, of course, Tommy will be seen on a regular basis throughout his life.

THE INTERVENTION

The recording of the intervention gave rise to most problems for the authors. Numerous attempts were made before a final decision on a format was reached which would be as simple and concise as possible. It was eventually decided to keep the intervention on the page facing the short- and long-term goals and the dates for evaluation (Fig. 3.4.1, p. 27). In this way there was no repetition in writing the headings of the activities of living. Continuation sheets (Figs 3.4.2 and 3.4.3, pp. 28-29) were superimposed on the original intervention sheet as required. It was very difficult to adjust to the idea of dividing the intervention into the categories of the activities of living for recording purposes. This was perhaps because it was so different from previous practice and because it seemed necessary at times to make what appeared to be unnatural divisions. For example, on 13th October the patient's mother was interviewed and various topics were discussed. This would normally be recorded as one entry but, using the intervention form, entries had to be made under three different categories: maintaining a safe environment, communicating, and eating and drinking.

It was decided that two charts already used in the ward were required in addition to those already described. These two charts are the Insulin Prescription Chart which is self-explanatory (Fig. 3.5, p. 30) and the Urinalysis and Blood Analysis Chart (Fig. 3.6, p. 31). In practical terms, the nurses and doctors found it convenient to have the data on these two charts readily available, and a series of findings seen at a glance on one sheet. These were kept at the nurses' station.

Discussion on the use of the model

After consideration, it was felt necessary to keep the record of diabetic education separate from the day-to-day ward report while, of course, being available to ward staff. There were two reasons for this. Firstly, the nurse concerned with education sees the patient over a long period of time, both as an inpatient and as an outpatient, and therefore wanted to have a record which would reflect progress as simply as possible. Secondly, the educational programme can be visualised as a separate entity in the overall care of the patient. Moreover while in this particular nursing study the care from the ward staff was fairly straightforward, on many occasions the patient might require treatment for ketoacidosis or infection at the same time as he is receiving his education. On those occasions the records of the ward staff would be much fuller.

Since the specialist nurse in the Diabetic Clinic has always spent a lot of time getting to know each new patient, the use of the activities of living did not necessarily give her more information than she previously acquired. However, the recording of this information in the activities of living framework produced a much more informative assessment and subsequent record of nursing activity than was formerly available.

This was also the reaction of the nurses in the ward,

particularly the learners who read the nursing study; they were enthusiastic about the presentation. It was noticeable that the learners did not appear to have the difficulties experienced by the authors in grasping the idea of dividing the nursing intervention into the categories of the activities of living. One student pointed out that this format would, in fact, make it easier to determine the patient's progress in any particular area, as well as give an overall profile.

From the point of view of nurse education, the learners would be able to use the records to discover how to tackle the educational programme for a patient (self-learning is exciting and effective). Also, the effect that diabetes has on a person's everyday activities would become more apparent and the need for the nurse to be aware of the patient and his family's normal habits would be obvious. If this type of record were available, a clinical teacher could help the learner to plan the nursing around the problems described.

Since nurses have a responsibility for health education, the model for nursing certainly permits the detection of those areas requiring planned help. For example, if the patient in this nursing study had had a poor standard of personal hygiene, this would have had to receive attention because of the diabetic patient's susceptibility to skin infection. After all, the activities of living are related to, and important for, maintaining a healthy life.

In addition, the model should help the nurse to involve the patient in the plan because she has noted what he can do for himself, and the contribution that can come from the family. This involvement is important for any patient but is particularly so for the diabetic who must take lifelong responsibility for the care of his own condition, and whose co-operation (with that of his family) is therefore imperative.

Having used the model for nursing with one patient, the question must be asked whether it would be practicable to use it with everyone. Obviously it is a very different matter to spend an unlimited amount of time with one patient for the purposes of a nursing study from having to deal with the normal number of patients seen each day in circumstances where time is at a premium.

Taking this into account, it is the opinion of the authors that the model could be used with all patients, provided it is adapted to the individual clinical area. In the area described, for example, there is a specialist nurse who is working constantly with diabetic patients; she sees the patients herself throughout the educational programme and, for many of the patients, the goals are similar. In these circumstances, to write a full list of short- and long-term goals and a detailed intervention for every patient would be unnecessary. Instead a précis could be made of the goals on a standardised form and

only sufficient information given about the intervention to allow other members of staff to follow the patient's progress. Biographical details, the initial assessment and a statement of problems would be required as in this study, as would an assessment to evaluate whether the patient is ready to take over his own care at home. In this way the amount of documentation could be substantially reduced while retaining the benefits of the model.

It is not suggested that this particular adaptation would necessarily be suitable for other areas. Where a person who has diabetes is being educated in a general ward by several members of nursing staff, some of whom may not be so familiar with diabetes, it would be necessary to keep a fuller list of goals in the nursing plan and to give more details of intervention. Nevertheless, with thought, it should be possible to preserve the advantages of the model while keeping the documentation to a minimum in many situations.

It must be emphasised that it took considerable time and energy (and we were well motivated) to adapt our thinking to the model and to apply it in practice. This should not be forgotten by others wishing to use this method. It was very important to refer frequently to *The Elements of Nursing* and to have a thorough knowledge of the actual ALs as described there.

Conclusion

The Committee on Nursing Report (1972) claims as fundamental to the educational system, acceptance of responsibility for teaching by all qualified staff in the clinical situation. There must be a direct relationship between the teaching in college and the teaching in the ward, clinic and community settings. The authors would conclude that the model for nursing can be used both in the classroom and in the practice area and would function, additionally, as the link between education and practice in nursing by involving qualified staff in teaching.

The method of documentation presented gives an accurate record of nursing activities, a safe platform from which to practise, and a method for learning. But more than that, it provides information from which a body of knowledge can accumulate regarding the educational needs of the patient, in this instance a patient with diabetes mellitus.

Never lose sight of the role your particular subject has within the great performance of the tragi-comedy of human life . . .
If you cannot — in the long run — tell everyone what you have been doing, your doing has been worthless.

Schrödinger

Figures to this chapter start on page 22.

Patient Assessment Form

Date of admission 7 Oct.

Date of assessment 8 Oct.

Surname McIntosh

Forenames Thomas

Male	✓
Female	

Age 15 yrs.

Date of birth

(Single)/Married/Widowed

Other

Prefers to be addressed as

Tommy

Address of usual residence

15 Glenlivit Road.

Type of accommodation Council flat, 3 apartment with bathroom.

Family/Others at this residence Parents and older brother.

Next of kin

Name John McIntosh

Relationship Father

Address S/A

Tel. no. 725 6812

Significant others

Relatives/Dependents

Helpers

Visitors

Occupation Schoolboy.

Religious beliefs and relevant practices R/C

Patient's perception of current health status Has known for some time that something was wrong because of polyuria and tiredness. Knows very little about diabetes as yet.

Reason for admission/referral Stabilisation of diabetes and education of patient and his family.

Medical diagnosis Juvenile onset diabetes mellitus.

Past medical history Motor cycle accident a year ago. No other illnesses of note.

Allergies nil.

Significant life crises nil.

Fig. 3.1 Patient Assessment Form: biographical and health data

Assessment of Activities of Living

Date

AL | Usual routines:
what he/she can and cannot do independently

Patient's problems
(actual/potential)
(p)= potential

● Maintaining
a safe
environment

● Communicating

● Breathing

● Eating and
drinking

● Eliminating

● Personal
cleansing and
dressing

● Controlling
body
temperature

● Mobilising

● Working
and playing

● Expressing
sexuality

● Sleeping

● Dying

Assessment of Activities of Living : Assessment ①

Date 8 Oct.

AL	Usual routines: what he/she can and cannot do independently	Patient's problems (actual/potential) (p)= potential
● Maintaining a safe environment	Independent till now.	● Lack of knowledge of diabetes on part of Tommy and his family.
● Communicating	Intelligent boy. Easy to chat to.	● (P) May feel strange in ward situation.
● Breathing	Normal.	
● Eating and drinking	Healthy appetite. Eats lots of sweets. Recently drinking 6 bottles lemonade daily.	● Lack of knowledge of how diabetes affects eating habits. ● (P) Very "sweet tooth."
● Eliminating	Recent polyuria – Improved since starting insulin yesterday.	
● Personal cleansing and dressing	Clean and tidy. Worried about spots on forehead. No trouble with feet.	● Worried about spots on forehead. ● Unaware of precautions he should take; especially regarding his feet.
● Controlling body temperature	Normal.	
● Mobilising	Normal.	
● Working and playing	4 th. year at school – "O" levels soon. Teachers have complained recently that he is lazy. Keen footballer – Played every day till recently. Knows younger boy at school who has diabetes	● Lack of energy. ● Lack of knowledge about effect of exercise on diabetic control
● Expressing sexuality	Seems well adjusted. He feels that he is very much younger than other inpatients.	
● Sleeping	Broken nights of late because of polyuria. Feels very tired.	● Tiredness
● Dying		

Fig. 3.2 Patient Assessment Form: assessment of ALs. First, second and third assessments

Assessment ②

Date 13 Oct.

	Outstanding problems

Has good grasp of what diabetes is.
Can self-inject safely and confidently.
Can test blood for glucose and understands
how to use results to adjust insulin. Can
recognise hypoglycaemia and hyperglycaemia.
Mother has also reasonable grasp of these things

● (P) May find it
difficult to carry
out regular
injections and
blood tests in
home situation.

Has friendly relationship with staff and
other patients. Tommy and mother
have good relationship.

Both Tommy and mother have good
grasp of diet.

● (P) May find it
difficult to resist
sweets and keep
mealtimes regular

No polyuria

Still has spots on forehead

Has a lot more energy. Knows in theory
how to make allowances for exercise
by adjusting   diet or insulin.

normal

Assessment ③

Date 20 Oct.

	Outstanding problems

Has now been home for a week. No
problems with injections. No
hypoglycaemia so far. Blood tests have
been within normal limits and tally
with test done at sideroom.

Back to school yesterday – everyone
there had already heard he has
diabetes and he did not mind too much.
Teachers had been very surprised to
hear about it.

Managing to keep to carbohydrate allowance
so far but is hungry in evenings –
increased his allowance today by 20 g.
So far he has refused all sweets.

No polyuria

Realises that, being back at school, he
may need to reduce insulin dosage
because of using more energy. Has been
playing football every day since discharge
and remembered to take extra to eat beforehand.

Nursing Plan

Activity of living	Short-term goals	Evaluation	Long-term goals	Evaluation
Maintaining a Safe Environment	Knows and understands before going home: • What diabetes is. • How to give insulin safely and confidently. • How to measure blood sugar and use it as a guide to diabetic control. • How to recognise and treat hypoglycaemia • What hyperglycaemia is, and when medical help is required to deal with it. • How to acquire and care for equipment. Family should also know these things.	13/10/	Accepts diabetes as an inconvenience which he controls while leading a normal life. Maintains good control and avoids complications of diabetes.	
Communicating	Feels happy and relaxed in the ward. Feels free to ask questions and discuss his condition.	13/10/	Feels free to ask for advice or help.	
Eating and Drinking	Has enough to eat to satisfy his appetite and allow normal growth. Both he and his mother understand need for carbohydrate control and can fit his dietary needs into family meal pattern. Knows how to cope with illness and special occasions.	13/10/	Eats a well balanced, carbohydrate controlled diet. Confident in fitting all kinds of carbohydrate foods into meals and in coping with unusual circumstances.	
Personal Cleansing and Dressing	Spots on forehead should clear. Feels reassured that this is a common adolescent problem. Knows how to care for feet.	13/10/	Takes good care of feet.	
Working and Playing	Feels fit and well. Understands how exercise affects diabetic control and how to allow for this.	13/10/	Performs work of his choice. Confidently takes any exercise he likes.	
Sleeping	Plenty of rest for next few days	13/10/	Should sleep well.	

Fig. 3.3 Nursing plan: goals and evaluation

Nursing Intervention

Date 7 Oct.

Admitted to ward from diabetic clinic.
Gave his first dose of insulin with help
before tea.
Had introductory chat about what diabetes
is & how symptoms arise.
Requires 6 hourly urinalysis for glucose
& ketones.
Requires observation for signs of hypoglycaemia

Introduced to ward staff & patients, told how
long he was likely to be in hospital, & the
examinations & tests he would be having. Sister
spoke to his mother & arranged a time for her to
come to ward for education.

Given a sugar - free meal & a supply of
saccharin to add to drinks
Advised about what to eat and drink
meantime

Date 8 Oct.

Managed before breakfast injection with
minimal help.
Learned how to draw up & measure insulin.
Discussed fact that he will always have
diabetes.
Drew up & injected evening dose of insulin
by himself.

Was given a booklet to read about diabetes
in his spare time.

Dietitian met Tommy & took diet history.
From this she estimated his carbohydrate need
as 300 g per day.
He learned about the different kinds of food
there are and which ones affect his diabetes.
Was given a basic diet sheet.

Advised to keep forehead clean & comb hair
back from it.

Discussed how diabetes might affect school
life & job prospects.

Fig. 3.4.1 Nursing plan: intervention

Nursing Intervention

Date 9 Oct.	Date 12 Oct.
managing injections well. Discussed different strengths of insulin, times of injection, rotation of sites. Discussed need for a balance between insulin dosage and carbohydrate intake. Mother interviewed along with Tommy – discussed what diabetes is, how it will affect Tommy at home. Mother had heard about "comas" – we talked about hypo and hyperglycaemic comas.	Giving injections confidently and safely Discussed hypoglycaemia – causes, prevention and treatment. Hyperglycaemia – when medical help is required. "Boiled up" glass syringe, discussed care of equipment, where to get supplies, disposal of used syringes and needles. Learned how to use blood testing strips and how to use results of these to adjust insulin dosage
Tommy said he does not intend to tell school friends about his diabetes. He has not yet read booklets given to him – encouraged to do so at weekend. Mother was given similar booklets to read at home.	Spent half an hour with a boy who has had diabetes for 14 years and is well adjusted to it. Indicated that his father is a heavy drinker. Has obviously spent time reading material given to him over the weekend and is beginning to come to terms with the changes he will need to make when he gets home.
Dietitian discussed with Tommy and mother need for regular carbohydrate intake, times of meals, diabetic products, what to do if feeling hungry between meals. He feels he is getting plenty to eat at present.	Discussed with dietitian relationship of illness, exercise and hypoglycaemia to diet, also how to incorporate occasional sweet and manufactured foods into diet. He is progressing well in understanding the diet. Had eaten several bars of diabetic chocolate on Saturday – despite warnings of effects of too much sorbitol – had bout of diarrhoea as a result.
Encouraged to be dressed in own clothes and go out for walks over the weekend.	Discussed need to take extra carbohydrate or less insulin before exercise particularly with regard to physical education at school and football in the evenings. Feeling well and full of energy. Has caught up on lost sleep.

Fig. 3.4.2 Nursing plan: intervention (contd)

Nursing Intervention

Date 13 Oct.	Date 14 Oct.
Had an induced hypoglycaemic attack this morning. He recognised the symptoms and these were reversed with a sweet drink. Revised causes, prevention and treatment of hypoglycaemia. Revised all topics covered last week and discussed insulin dosage if sick, visiting dentist and immunisations. mother interviewed – has read all material given to her and is coming to terms with Tommy having diabetes. Discussed care of equipment, injections, hypoglycaemia. She stayed to watch Tommy give his evening injection.	Given supply of equipment for home. Given card to carry with him and note of insulin dose on it. Given telephone number to call in case of problems. Asked to come back to sideroom on 16/10/
Discussed with mother when Tommy should go back to school and gave her a leaflet for the school staff.	Discharged home late morning.
Dietitian revised diet with Tommy and mother. Discussed alcohol with Tommy – said he wanted nothing to do with it and did not want to know what he could or could not drink – advised him to come back if he ever changed his mind.	
Chiropodist discussed care of feet and examined feet.	

Fig. 3.4.3   Nursing plan: intervention (contd)

INSULIN PRESCRIPTION CHART

Date of birth _____ Hospital no. _____

First name _Thomas_   Surname _McIntosh_

Address _15 Glenlivit Road_   Sex/Marital status _____

Occupation _____

Hospital _____ Wd/Dept _____ Consultant _____

DATE	TYPE	DOSE	ROUTE	TIME ORDERED FOR	ORDERED BY	TIME GIVEN	GIVEN BY	CHECKED BY
7/10	MIXTARD	28 u	SC	BT	J. Brown	4.40 pm	Patient	E.M. Howie
8/10	MIXTARD	24 u	SC	BB	J. Brown	8.30 am	Patient	E.M. Howie
8/10	MIXTARD	20 u	SC	BT	J. Brown	5.30 pm	Patient	E.M. Howie
9/10	MIXTARD	20 u	SC	BB	J. Brown	8.35 am	Patient	E.M. Howie
9/10	MIXTARD	20 u	SC	BT	J. White	5.15 pm	Patient	E.M. Howie
10/10	MIXTARD	20 u	SC	BB	J. White	8 am	Patient	R. Black
10/10	MIXTARD	20 u	SC	BT	J. White	5.30 pm	Patient	P. Grey
11/10	MIXTARD	20 u	SC	BB	J. White	8 am	Patient	P. Grey
11/10	MIXTARD	20 u	SC	BT	J. Brown	5.20 pm	Patient	R. Black
12/10	MIXTARD	20 u	SC	BB	J. Brown	8.30 am	Patient	E.M. Howie
12/10	MIXTARD	20 u	SC	BT	J. Brown	5.15 pm	Patient	E.M. Howie
13/10	MIXTARD	24 u	SC	BB	J. Brown	8.30 am	Patient	E.M. Howie
	VELOSULIN	8 u	SC					
13/10	MIXTARD	20 u	SC	BT	J. Brown	5 pm	Patient	E.M. Howie
14/10	MIXTARD	24 u	SC	BB	J. Brown	8.35 am	Patient	E.M. Howie

Fig. 3.5 Insulin prescription chart (form already in use in ward)

Date of birth _____   Hospital no. _____

First name *Thomas*   Surname *McIntosh*

Address *15 Glenlivit Road*   Sex/Marital status _____

_____   Occupation _____

Hospital _____ Wd/Dept _____   Consultant _____

No. 1208

Date		7/10				8/10				9/10				10/10				11/10				12/10				13/10			
Weight																													
Hypoglycaemic Agent Given																													
Time		BB	BL	BT	10PM	BB	BL	BT	10PM	BB	BL	BT	10PM	BB	BL	BT	10PM	BB	BL	BT	10PM	BB	BL	BT	10PM	BB	BL	BT	10PM
Glycosuria (Clinitest)	Red/Orange =2%																												
	Yellow =1%																												
	Green =0.5%																												
	Blue =0%																												
Ketonuria (Acetest)	Strong =+++																												
	Moderate =++																												
	Trace = +																												
	Negative = 0																												
Blood Sugar m. mol/l				30		8.1	9.6	5.4	6.9	6.6	18.8	7.0										10	8.5	15.8	14.2	9	6.5	12.1	7.2
Diet No. of Calories and Carbohydrate Content																													

Date		14/10																											
Weight																													
Hypoglycaemic Agent Given																													
Time		BB	BL	BT	10PM	BB	BL	BT	10PM	BB	BL	BT	10PM	BB	BL	BT	10PM	BB	BL	BT	10PM	BB	BL	BT	10PM	BB	BL	BT	10PM
Glycosuria (Clinitest)	Red/Orange =2%																												
	Yellow =1%																												
	Green =0.5%																												
	Blue =0%																												
Ketonuria (Acetest)	Strong =+++																												
	Moderate = ++																												
	Trace = +																												
	Negative = 0																												
Blood Sugar m. mol/l																													
Diet No. of Calories and Carbohydrate Content																													

SLIDING SCALE SOLUBLE INSULIN

IF URINE   RED/ORANGE   (2%)   GIVE .... UNITS

IF URINE   YELLOW   (1%)   GIVE .... UNITS

IF URINE   GREEN   (0.5%) GIVE .... UNITS

IF URINE   BLUE   (0.0%) GIVE .... UNITS

IF ACETONE PRESENT GIVE .... EXTRA UNITS

N.B. ROUTINE HYPOGLYGAEMIC AGENTS PRESCRIBED ON DRUG KARDEX

NOTE — BB = 30 mins before breakfast

BL = 30 mins before lunch

BT = 30 mins before tea

Fig. 3.6 Urinalysis and blood analysis chart (form already in use in ward)

4

A study in a surgical ward

using the model for nursing

Elizabeth M. Stewart and Heather C. Strachan

Ward background

In the busy surgical ward selected for this project the nursing staff had for some time been using a 'mini' form of the nursing process; each patient on admission had a brief nursing history taken, usually by one of the student nurses, and the ward sister would then start a nursing care plan which was kept in a readily accessible central Kardex. The headings under which nursing care was ordered followed fairly closely those used by Collingwood (1975), i.e., personal hygiene and basic needs; mobilisation; observations; technical care; diet; treatment and investigations; special needs and future plans. Although most of the nursing planning was done by the ward sisters, the student nurses were encouraged to contribute suggestions for planning and for giving nursing care.

An important point is that during initial discussions of this project the student nurse, a senior student close to registration, made it clear to the other project member, the nurse teacher, that she considered the standard of nursing in the ward was high and that the documentation used was adequate in helping achieve this, and although willing to participate in this project she saw no need for any real change from the traditional nursing approach. Her reaction to using the activities of living (AL) model in the application of the nursing process is described below.

Preparation for the project

First, however, a brief description of some of the preparatory thinking is appropriate. We saw no difficulties in using the Patient Assessment Form: biographical and health data (Fig. 4.1, p. 38) and the Patient Assessment Form: assessment of ALs (Fig. 4.2, p. 39) and we were required to use problem-oriented nursing plans which we wanted, if possible, to reflect the activities of living approach to nursing. Because it was unrealistic to expect that a student nurse new to problem-documentation would find it easy to write by hand all the many problems which could be anticipated, it was decided to reduce that commitment by utilising the concept of 'usual' problems as described by Mayers (1978). She maintains that patients with the same diagnosis have more similarities than differences, and 'usual' problems are those which are predictable or frequently occurring. Standard nursing care plans, each containing the usual problems relevant to a given situation, can then be developed and are instantly available for use when required.

So using the AL framework, usual problems which are associated with the preoperative and postoperative periods of surgery were identified and two forms were devised — Standard Preoperative Nursing Care Plan (Fig. 4.3, pp. 40-41) and Standard Postoperative Nursing Care Plan (Fig. 4.4, pp. 42-43). This exercise provided the student with a valuable opportunity for practising problem-oriented thinking and recording, in fact that is why these Plans were produced in such detail. Commonly these activities are documented as simple checklists of routine instructions; and indeed our Plans could be seen as an elaboration of a checklist.

They were retained in this way, however, at the request of the ward sister from the surgical area. When asked to check the content of the Standard Plans, she emphasised their helpfulness in illustrating the reasons for, and the importance of preoperative and postoperative nursing activities to students and pupil nurses during their early surgical experience.

The problems common to preoperative surgical patients were identified without difficulty within the AL framework; postoperative problems however were less straightforward. Some could be associated readily with more than one AL; a simple example was the temporary dependence in washing and hygiene activities, but finally it was decided that the problem was basically one of 'mobilising' rather than of 'personal cleansing and dressing'. Some problems were more difficult to categorise; the problem of pain can affect functioning in each of the twelve ALs, but it was thought that it ought to be assessed also in terms of how the patient felt about the pain. So pain was not categorised within one of the 12 ALs. Similarly the potential problem of haemorrhage, internal or external, is one which no nurse responsible for postoperative care could possibly ignore, and which too could affect all of the ALs, but it had no obvious association with any one heading. So haemorrhage too was left uncategorised.

In order to provide some measures to help with evaluation, we set out in the two Standard Nursing Care Plans not only goals, but also goal criteria, and once nursing intervention was listed the three columns on the right-hand side of the plan were to be used as follows:

Evaluate: The date or deadline time was the predicted time by which it was anticipated the goal would be reached. In addition check times for reporting progress were also stated.

Item discontinued: this provided a means of discontinuing before the stated deadline individual nursing interventions, while continuing others.

Problem resolved: the date when the goal was reached and all related nursing intervention was discontinued.

So before the patient was admitted, Standard Nursing Care Plans (preoperative and postoperative) had been formulated and typed, and indeed a copy of each could have been used for any patient who was to have surgery.

A hand-written *Individual* Nursing Care Plan (Fig. 4.5, pp. 44-45) would contain all actual and potential problems not already identified on the *Standard* Plans.

We saw defining nursing discharge goals as part of the discipline of the exercise and since the frame of reference was dependence/independence within each AL, a simple chart was developed, the AL Status Indicator (Fig. 4.6, p. 46) on which the patient's changing — or unchanging — status within each AL could be recorded. The more serious use of the chart, however, was to reinforce the daily focus of assessment of the patient's problems in terms of ALs.

It was decided that the normal ward routine of writing a Progress/Evaluation Record (Fig. 4.7, p. 47) three times a day, at 8 a.m., 12 noon and 8 p.m. was to be followed but the reports were to be statements concerning the patient's problems relating to ALs and were to be made according to the predetermined check-times or deadlines on the nursing plans. In addition if any special procedures had been performed these were to be reported along with the patient's response. We wanted, at the end of the patient's stay in hospital, to have a record of the patient's response to the nursing care.

We had by now done a considerable amount of thinking and planning and we were ready to start. In the next part of the chapter, the student nurse gives an account of how she carried out the nursing study.

The nursing study

PREPARATION PRIOR TO ADMISSION

Before Mrs Rogers' admission I, the student nurse, read her case notes and transferred some of the information from them to the Patient Assessment Form: biographical and health data (Fig. 4.1, p. 38). This meant I would not have to repeat questions she would be asked at reception such as address and next of kin. The notes also gave me information about her past medical and surgical history and the circumstances leading up to her planned admission for an elective cholecystectomy.

As I did not want other patients to see that Mrs Rogers was receiving any special nursing attention a single room was made ready for her, which also ensured privacy for the assessment. In preparation for the assessment interview I had drawn up a short list of questions in areas which I felt were likely to be appropriate and of value to nurses in looking after such a patient admitted for elective surgery.

Although I was quite happy with the existing system of patient care and documentation, I was looking forward to using the nursing process and the new model with the activities of living approach.

ASSESSMENT ON ADMISSION

When Mrs Rogers arrived I introduced myself and explained that I was doing a special nursing study with some new documentation using a new approach to planning nursing care while she was in hospital. She said she would be very pleased to help and throughout her stay showed a great interest in the project.

The Patient Assessment Form: biographical and health data (Fig. 4.1, p. 38) was the first form I filled in. I felt this was a good form. It had all the basic information needed for the nurses and gave a good outline of the home background which is helpful among other things in planning the patient's discharge from hospital. I thought that the questions were adequate and had no difficulty in asking them. The significant life crises was a little different as I felt I could not directly ask about this, but hoped that as we talked or possibly at a future time any significant problem would be revealed. But Mrs Rogers did not appear to have any such problems.

Before starting to assess the ALs I asked Mrs Rogers how she felt generally about coming in to hospital. This question gave her the opportunity to express how she felt at that moment and showed her that I was interested in her and hopefully it would also help her to relax. Her reply gave me an idea of the type of person she was, and how she would cope in hospital. She appeared very well organised and at this point she spoke of her 30-year-old handicapped son. Although her sister, whom her son knew well, was to look after him, she was apprehensive about his reaction to enforced separation. This I identified as a problem.

In using the Patient Assessment Form: assessment of ALs (Fig. 4.2, p. 39) I did not follow the order of ALs as listed, as some questions followed naturally after others.

As far as the twelve ALs were concerned, I thought that there was such a variety of headings that there was likely to be a place to put any particular piece of information. However, I did find a little difficulty in classifying a few of the items as some could be placed under two or three headings, e.g., Mrs Rogers needed to wear glasses all the time as her eye-sight was not very good. This could be a problem if she did not have her glasses with her and could therefore be placed under 'communicating', 'mobilising' and 'maintaining a safe environment'. Mrs Rogers had a good pair of glasses and as long as she wore them there was no problem.

I found no difficulty in asking questions but I did feel there was not a great deal of space on the Patient Assessment Form for large writing or for much information to be noted. Not all of the ALs were, of course, relevant to Mrs Rogers. And some information such as temperature and urinalysis were noted on the form but this was duplication of information as these were also recorded elsewhere. On the other hand, there seemed no obvious place to include a note of the pulse or blood pressure which are equally routinely checked on admission by the nurse.

The assessment interview took approximately 40 minutes. This may seem rather a long time and hardly realistic on a busy ward with five or six admissions daily. But I believe the time would be reduced if I were accustomed to this type of assessment; it would become easier and therefore quicker. Also approximately 15–20 minutes of that time were used to explain about the theatre routine for her operation the next day. On our Standard Preoperative Nursing Care Plan (Fig. 4.3, pp. 40-41) we had identified the 'usual' potential problem of preoperative anxiety. I was therefore alert to the possibility of this being present and indeed Mrs Rogers admitted that she was worried about the operation. Therefore I took the opportunity to explain what would happen to her and she did appear to be more relaxed after that.

I felt that using the AL approach was helpful in a nursing assessment. It ensured that the patient was looked at as a whole person. Mrs Rogers' normal habits, likes and dislikes were discussed and could be adapted for her stay in hospital and any areas of potential or actual problems could be identified early and suitable action planned.

There was an enthusiastic reaction from other nurses on the ward who liked the Patient Assessment Form. Communication between staff regarding information about Mrs Rogers was good. By reading this form new nurses to the ward were able to learn a little more about the patient than they normally would have known. For example they were made aware that Mrs Rogers had a handicapped son. This meant she was able to talk openly about him without any embarrassment. Although it was not realised in the initial assessment, Mrs Rogers stated later that she had been a little worried and apprehensive about how people would react to her son's loud voice. This however did not even become an embarrassment because all the nurses were interested in hearing about him and when he visited she was happy to see him accepted. Mrs Rogers actually stated that she felt much more welcome than on her previous admission to hospital.

IDENTIFICATION OF THE PROBLEMS

After completing the nursing assessment I made my list of potential and actual problems of which she had very few. As already mentioned I identified her anxiety about her handicapped son's reaction to her hospitalisation as an actual problem.

Mrs Rogers' overweight was also identified as a problem; she had had previous diet sheets but had 'dieted' unsuccessfully. We briefly discussed what had to be done but decided to postpone any real intervention or teaching until after surgery.

One item worthy of a special mention under the heading 'eating and drinking' was occasional indigestion, not surprising in view of her diagnosis. I did not feel it was necessary to document it as a problem because Mrs Rogers had coped well with it and did not herself see it as a problem. She preferred to suffer occasional discomfort rather than resort to medication. She would also only be having one meal preoperatively and would then be prepared for her operation which would hopefully resolve this particular difficulty.

She usually smoked 20 cigarettes a day and did not foresee any difficulty about stopping while she was in hospital. The habit of smoking was not seen by her as a problem, so I did not identify it as such, but an associated higher than usual risk of postoperative chest infection was recorded later because of this.

An Individual Nursing Care Plan (Fig. 4.5, pp. 44-45) was then started with the identified problems entered under AL headings. No difficulty was found with their classification and I used a fresh page of nursing care plan for each problem.

FORMULATION OF DISCHARGE GOALS

Normally the hope is that our patients will go home fit after a successful operation. We do not consciously think about patient or nursing goals, so formulating discharge goals was a good exercise since it made me work out just what we were aiming for from the nurses' and patient's points of view. I wrote Mrs Rogers' discharge goals on a separate form but since this is not reproduced here, the goals are stated below.

On discharge Mrs Rogers would:
1. be independent in all activities of living
2. verbalize the importance of, and express willingness to continue, a weight reduction diet
3. express understanding of instructions for a convalescent period with regard to exercise, rest and an outpatient appointment.

I doubt if I would normally have felt it necessary — or indeed my responsibility — to have planned a patient education session regarding Mrs Rogers' weight had I not been made to think of discharge goals and it could be especially useful for highlighting the less obvious but nevertheless important areas of useful patient-teaching for patients with chronic illness or disability.

PLANNING THE NURSING CARE

Most of all I enjoyed using the problem-oriented nursing care plans. I found that the problems listed on the Standard Preoperative Nursing Care Plan and also on the Standard Postoperative Nursing Care Plan (Figs 4.3 and 4.4, pp. 40-43) were appropriate as we had anticipated, and the time saved by using them was invaluable as I did tend to spend rather a long time working out what I should write for each problem on the Individual Nursing Care Plan. Only one postoperative potential problem — nausea — became an actual problem and had to be transferred to Mrs Rogers' Individual Nursing Care Plan in order that the now real problem could be dealt with by appropriately altered intervention. The potential problem of chest infection was repeated on the Individual Nursing Care Plan as I felt that Mrs Rogers with her high abdominal incision, and history of smoking, required rather more nursing intervention than was ordered on the Standard Postoperative Nursing Care Plan.

Although the nursing care given pre-and postoperatively was not obviously different from the nursing care which she would have received anyway, having detailed nursing care plans meant that her nursing really was planned and ensured that her needs were met. I felt that the plans improved communication between shifts and were good teaching aids for students and pupil nurses.

In order to make communication easier still and because the plans were unfamiliar to most of the staff I used a 'nursing order' sheet which was kept at the foot of Mrs Rogers' bed and on that the nursing intervention was pencilled in when ordered, and erased when discontinued. This temporarily duplicated the record of nursing intervention which could have been found on the Standard and Individual Nursing Care Plans, but it did ensure that whoever attended Mrs Rogers knew what had to be done.

Throughout the preoperative and postoperative periods I continued to use the AL mode of thinking and as a reminder every day I used the AL Status Indicator (Fig. 4.6, p. 46) Charting was done on a daily basis as surgical patients are generally in hospital for a short time and their dependence after surgery can change rapidly compared with that of many medical patients.

The AL Status Indicator was simple to fill in and I found no difficulties in identifying problems through thinking of the ALs. Although initially I anticipated that any decrease in independence as shown on the Indicator would be reflected by an identified problem on the nursing care plan, this was not exactly the case. For example on the theatre day although 'working and playing' was nearer dependence than independence I felt that it was not necessary to record this as a problem on the nursing care plan. However it was a good visual chart of dependence/independence for the nursing and medical staff.

The AL Status Indicator was kept with the assessment forms and nursing care plans at the nurses' station. I would have preferred to have had it by the bed-side and in Mrs Rogers' case there would have been no difficulties, but if it were used more generally the 'expressing sexuality' and 'dying' categories could require some tricky explanations.

REPORTING PROGRESS AND PATIENT OUTCOME

Looking at Mrs Rogers' nursing Kardex reports from a previous admission, all I found were comments such as 'slept well' or 'usual day' or 'up and about'. This told me nothing about her care or her progress. The system was different this time because I had to think about Mrs Rogers' actual and potential problems at the previously decided checktimes and deadlines. This made sense in a Progress Evaluation Record (Fig. 4.7, p. 47) and was in fact a more structured extension of the system used already on the ward whereby nursing intervention relating to a specific aspect of care is recorded in the Kardex and commented upon by the nurse responsible.

On the whole the system worked whereby I reported on the problems at the predetermined check-times and deadlines and I did think it useful to include a time limit for each goal. But this meant that two problems, pain and insomnia, which ceased to be problems several days before their deadlines, continued to be unnecessarily reported. More flexible 'deadlines' could perhaps be used, especially on Standard Nursing Care Plans.

Reporting under AL headings was straightforward with the two unclassified problems reported under their own headings. All normal ward documentation continued to be used during this project, so I was the only nurse who completed the new reports. As a result some of them were inevitably written retrospectively following evenings, mornings or days off.

Although overall there appears to be more documentation it did not require a great deal more writing than the present system and I feel that it is an improvement due to the greater detail recorded.

Mrs Rogers made an uneventful and good recovery and on the tenth day was discharged home. Before her departure she expressed how much she had enjoyed her stay and how much she had appreciated all the care. Although we normally have no further contact with most outpatients, Mrs Rogers visited the ward when she returned for an outpatient appointment four weeks later, to show off her new slim 70 kg figure.

Conclusions about the use of the model for nursing

It is difficult, on the basis of a single nursing study carried out by a single student, to have anything other than very tentative conclusions but there is no doubt that the reaction of the student to using the AL mode of thinking in nursing the patient was positive. She liked it, finding it sensible, and with a few exceptions suitable and easy to use. And, as noted already, it acted as a stimulus for her to take, and accept, a wider view of nursing's contribution to a patient's care.

But in spite of her enthusiasm and the daily use of the AL Status Indicator, admittedly a very blunt tool, she does confess to some difficulties in knowing how 'pure' her use of the AL approach actually was. A senior student, already with two months of surgical nursing experience in looking after patients having abdominal surgery, she was bound to have certain expectations of a patient's needs and care to be given. However this hardly matters except perhaps, in the case of the two unclassified problems, pain and potential haemorrhage. As both were predicted as 'usual' problems arising from non-defined 'surgery', the question arises as to whether having the predictive, i.e., Standard Nursing Care Plan inadvertently prevented a really fresh look being taken at the patient during her postoperative period. We do not know.

As it was, pain relief was part of the nursing intervention ordered in relation to breathing and sleeping. It was not included in the mobilising category, but could have been, to help cope with the pain part of the difficulty which patients have in starting ambulation. But would the inclusion of intervention to reduce pain in order to achieve goals in these three categories obviate the need to define postoperative pain as a patient's problem? In Mrs Rogers' case it probably would. Would the patient who has less limiting but painful surgery appreciate being given pain relief for reasons of sleep only? Pain may not always manifest itself in overt behaviour, and if the definition given by Hunt (1979) is used: 'Pain is whatever the patient says that it is', pain should be a 'communicating' problem.

Had the potential problem of haemorrhage become an actual problem to Mrs Rogers following the cholecystectomy, it would probably have occurred sometime during the first 24 postoperative hours, initially affecting her already restricted mobility and if it became severe, her other ALs. But even when related specifically to Mrs Rogers it does not fit readily into any one category.

So there are gaps in either our application or in the AL

model itself. These gaps were emphasised by our attempt to classify each problem under only *one* AL heading on the nursing care plans. In the normal working environment this classification would be seen as unnecessary; problems would stand alone and progress evaluation would be reported in relation to the problem. A too rigid application of the model therefore may well detract from its value. We rather think that the model may be of most benefit when used on admission, and on discharge of a patient. During a hospital stay involving surgery, in addition to the AL mode of thinking, appropriate application of professional knowledge related to surgical nursing — it matters not from which model — should be used.

The 'Patient Assessment Form: assessment of ALs' being semi-structured provides scope for the prepared and perceptive interviewer, but one small difficulty always exists with semi- or unstructured interview schedules — if comment about a certain aspect of the patient's functioning is seen not to be noted it is not easy to know whether indeed he has no difficulty or whether questions were asked at all in that area. Many nursing assessments will be done by student nurses and it is essential that they be given adequate guidance with some plan to follow in order that the interview is seen by the patient as relevant, and the collected information worthwhile for nursing.

In the U.S.A. where nursing care plans have been in use for much longer than in this country Stevens (1979) notes a continuing reluctance by many nurses to actually write anything on them. This may become a stimulus for computerising the plans, but for most hospitals that is in the distant future. At this point in time, if nursing plans are to be written and maintained by busy clinical nurses, account must be taken of limited time. The Nursing Care Plans used in this project were designed to detail some of the thinking behind the nursing, unnecessary for experienced nurses but a valuable exercise in a process of thinking by which a student nurse comes to understand what she is doing and why she is doing it.

Acknowledgement

The authors of this chapter would like to acknowledge the help given by Margaret Black, Nursing Officer, without whom the project could not have been undertaken.

REFERENCES

Collingwood M P 1975 The nursing care plan. Nursing Times 71 (12): 22
Hunt J M 1979 Protracted pain and nursing care. Nursing 2: 56
Mayers M G 1978 A systematic approach to the nursing care plan, 2nd edn. Appleton-Century-Crofts, New York, p 15
Stevens B J 1979 Why won't nurses write nursing care plans? In: Marriner A (ed) The nursing process, 2nd edn. Mosby, St Louis, p 115

Figures to this chapter start on page 38.

Patient Assessment Form

Date of admission 29/9   Date of assessment 29/9

Surname Rogers   Forenames Janet

Male		Age		Single/Married/Widowed	Prefers to be addressed as
Female	✓		53	Other Divorced	Mrs. Rogers

Date of birth

Address of usual residence   1 Nelson Street.

Type of accommodation   Semi-detached house.

Family/Others at this residence   Sister and son aged 30 (mentally handicapped).

Next of kin   Name Mary Smith   Address Same address.

                   Relationship Sister   Tel. no. 321 5865

Significant others   Relatives/Dependents 5 sisters all living nearby.

                      Helpers Sister who lives with Mrs. Rogers, helps with son.

                      Visitors Family and friends.

Occupation   Housewife

Religious beliefs and relevant practices Church of Scotland.

Patient's perception of current health status   Mrs Rogers has come into hospital to have her gall-bladder removed because of gall-stones. She hopes this will relieve her symptoms of heartburn and pai

Reason for admission/referral   List admission for a cholecystectomy.

Medical diagnosis   Pancreatitis and cholecystitis.

Past medical history   Tuberculosis – removal of kidney cyst (age 19)
                       D+C x 3 for polyps: bone biopsy

Allergies   none known | Significant life crises

Fig. 4.1   Patient Assessment Form: biographical and health data

Assessment of Activities of Living

Date 29/9

Patient's problems
(actual/potential)
(p)= potential

AL	Usual routines: what he/she can and cannot do independently	
● Maintaining a safe environment	Has mentioned a dislike of taking medication.	
● Communicating	Wears glasses at all times. She is a pleasant lady who is very open and easy to talk to. Generally anxious about coming into hospital and leaving her mentally handicapped son. He is being cared for by her sister.	● Anxiety about her son.
● Breathing	Smokes 20 cigarettes a day. Has a "wheeze" and becomes breathless on exertion. Has a slight cough.	● (P) Chest infection.
● Eating and drinking	Unable to eat a full meal or fatty foods. Recently she has been "picking" at her food. She occasionally suffers from dyspepsia after eating but refuses to consider medication and copes with the problem by taking small meals. Overweight and is concerned about this. Wt. 81.2 kg Ht. 1.626 m	● Overweight
● Eliminating	No problems with micturition. Urinalysis normal. Bowels move regularly each day. No aperients taken.	
● Personal cleansing and dressing	Personal cleanliness good. Smart well groomed lady. Prefers to have a bath as showers frighten her a little. Has her own teeth.	
● Controlling body temperature	Temperature 36.6°C on admission.	
● Mobilising	No problems with mobility. No aids required.	
● Working and playing	Enjoys reading and knitting. She spends a lot of time with her handicapped son.	
● Expressing sexuality	Post-menopausal.	
● Sleeping	Normally sleeps well.	
● Dying		

Fig. 4.2 Patient Assessment Form: assessment of ALs

STANDARD PREOPERATIVE NURSING CARE PLAN for patients having elective surgery

Name: *Mrs. Janet Rogers*   Date of admission: 29/9/

PROBLEM and cause(s)	GOAL and goal criterion/criteria	INTERVENTION	EVALUATE	DATES AND INITIALS ITEM DISCONTINUED	PROBLEM RESOLVED
Maintaining a safe environment					
Potential injury from or damage to: dentures, contact lenses, spectacles, hearing aid, jewellery, hair clips	No injury from or damage to prostheses or jewellery. *Criteria* Adequate preventive and protective measures are taken	• Remove jewellery, or tape wedding ring • Remove prostheses N.B. if hearing aid to be retained until after induction of anaesthesia, note this on 'Recovery Room and Postoperative Form' • Ensure that articles are kept in safe place while patient is in theatre	Before giving pre-med		N.M. 30 Sept.
Potential wrong patient or wrong operation due to: mixed up, identity or information	Correct patient goes to theatre with correct documentation. *Criteria* No mistakes are made	• Check name on 'Recovery Room and Postoperative Form' brought by porter • Check unit number • Check identiband • Check correct case record • Check correct X-rays	Morning of surgery		N.M. 30 Sept.
Communicating					
Potential anxiety due to: impending surgery/anaesthetic	No excessive anxiety. *Criteria* No signs of undue anxiety. States that anxiety is reduced	• Give opportunity to ask questions regarding surgery • Give information about: preparation in ward transfer to theatre induction of anaesthetic the recovery room anticipated pattern of postoperative care including IV infusion or drainage tubes pain and the availability of analgesia	At latest, day before surgery		N.M. 30 Sept.
Breathing					
Potential respiratory problems due to: regurgitation and aspiration of gastric contents while	Reduced risk of aspiration. *Criteria* Stomach known to be empty before anaesthetic given	• Fast for at least 4 hours before surgery	Morning of surgery		N.M. 30 Sept.

Problem	Goal / Criteria	Nursing action	Timing	Signature / Date
Potential incontinence of urine and faeces due to: loss of voluntary muscle control while unconscious	Reduced risk of incontinence *Criteria* Bladder and bowel are known to be empty before going to theatre	● Give suppositories or enema and have evidence of good bowel movement ● Ensure bladder is empty before pre-medication is given	Evening before surgery Morning of surgery	29 Sept. N.M. 30 Sept.
Personal cleansing, dressing *Potential* wound infection due to: bacteria from skin or clothing	Reduced risk of wound infection *Criteria* Skin is intact and smooth after preoperative shave Skin is clean after bath	● Shave areas appropriate to type of surgery ● Give bath ● Give bath ● Dress in clean cotton (hospital) gown and cap ● Strip and remake bed with clean linen for patient's return from bath	Evening before surgery Morning of surgery	H.S. 29 Sept. N.M. 30 Sept.
Mobilising *Potential* deep venous thrombosis due to: immobility	Reduced risk of deep venous thrombosis *Criteria* Appropriate preventive measures started	● Reinforce physiotherapist's teaching of leg and breathing exercises ● Unless contra-indicated, encourage mobility during preoperative period	Evening before surgery	H.S. 29 Sept.
Sleeping *Potential* insomnia due to: apprehension and strange environment	Refreshing sleep before surgery *Criteria* Observed to sleep for most of night States that she/he slept	● Ensure peaceful, quiet environment ● Check physical and emotional comfort of patient before she/he settles for sleep ● Give sedative if prescribed	Daily	N.M. 30 Sept.
Potential complications related to surgery and anaesthesia	Safe surgery and recovery	● If arising, report on INDIVIDUAL NURSING CARE PLAN		

Fig. 4.3 Standard Preoperative Nursing Care Plan

STANDARD POSTOPERATIVE NURSING CARE PLAN

Name: *Mrs Janet Rogers*   Time/Date return to ward: 12.30 pm. 30/9/

PROBLEM and cause(s)	GOAL and goal criterion/criteria	INTERVENTION	EVALUATE	DATES AND INITIALS ITEM DIS-CONTINUED	PROBLEM RESOLVED
Breathing *Potential* respiratory failure due to: Sensitivity to or incomplete reversal of anaesthetic agents	Adequate respiration *Criteria* Rate and depth of respiration remain within normal limits Good colour maintained	● Record respiratory rate and depth ½ hrly — 1 hrly — 2 hrly then 4 hrly as levels stabilise ● Observe colour	For 8 hrs post-op		H.S. 30 Sept.
Potential chest infection due to: Effects of anaesthesia and immobility	No chest infection *Criteria* No change in normal respiratory pattern No purulent sputum	● Prop up as conscious level/surgery will permit ● Encourage deep breathing and expectoration 2 hrly when awake ● Give adequate analgesia ● Start mobilising as soon as condition allows	12 noon until Day 2 post-op	Problem referred to individual A.&.P.	
Eating and drinking *Potential* nausea and vomiting due to: Effects of anaesthesia	No nausea or vomiting *Criteria* Able to take regulated amounts of fluid States that no nausea is present	● Avoid unnecessary movement ● Position comfortably ● Give anti-emetics as prescribed ● Give gradually increasing amounts of oral fluids as ordered and as tolerated	8 p.m. 8 a.m. 12 noon until 24 hrs post-op	Problem referred to individual A.b.P.	
Eliminating *Potential* retention of urine due to: Effects of surgery and anaesthesia	Normal micturition *Criteria* No undue bladder distension No undue bladder discomfort	● Offer urinal or bedpan within 6 hrs postoperatively ● If any difficulty: ● help into normal position for voiding unless contra-indicated ● provide privacy ● encourage by sound of running water ● encourage oral fluids unless contra-indicated ● Record amount and time of voiding ● Consider obtaining an order for neuromuscular drug or for catheterisation if above methods fail	8 p.m. 8 a.m. 12 noon until 24 hrs post-op		H.S. 1 Oct.
Personal cleansing and dressing *Potential* wound infection due to: Bacterial contamination and growth	No wound infection *Criteria* Good wound healing	● Wound care according to ward policy ● Aseptic technique if/when wound dressed	12 noon until wound is healed		H.S. 19 Oct.

Problem	Criteria	Nursing actions	Timing	Signature/Date
Potential deep venous thrombosis due to: Immobility/effects of surgery	No deep venous thrombosis *Criteria* No pain in leg(s) No swelling of leg(s) No otherwise unexplained pyrexia	● Remind patient not to lie with legs crossed ● Encourage leg and deep breathing exercises ● Start mobilisation as soon as able	12 noon until one week after mobility resumed	H.S. 10 Oct. H.S. 10 Oct.
Potential pressure sores due to: Immobility	Healthy intact pressure areas *Criteria* No redness No bruising No skin damage	● Change, or help patient to change position 2-4 hrly ● Consider potential benefit of aids e.g. sheepskin ● Keep skin dry; wash only for bathing or hygiene reasons	12 noon until Day 2 post-op	H.S. 2 Oct. H.S. 2 Oct. N.Ar. 4 Oct.
Reduced mobility due to: Effects of surgery	Independence in mobilising *Criteria* Able to get in and out of bed and walk without help Wash and groom self	● Give help with position changing in bed encouraging gradual self-movement ● Give help with washing and grooming encouraging gradual self-help ● Assist with and encourage increasing periods of ambulation	12 noon 8 p.m. until Day 4 post-op	N.Ar. 4 Oct.
Sleeping *Potential* insomnia due to: Pain Apprehension	Long periods of normal sleep during the night *Criteria* Observed to sleep for long periods States she has slept No evidence of undue tiredness	● Minimise number of disturbances by planned timing of interventions e.g. BP, position change ● Ensure peaceful, quiet environment ● Check physical and emotional comfort before settling for sleep ● Give analgesic or sedative if ordered	8 a.m. until discharge	Ar.B. 10 Oct.
Potential haemorrhage due to: Surgery	Early detection of haemorrhage *Criteria* Rising pulse rate Falling BP Increasing skin pallor Swelling near, or blood staining through wound dressing Undue restlessness Decreased response Oliguria	● Record pulse and BP ½ hrly — 1 hrly — 2 hrly then 4 hrly as levels stabilise ● Observe colour and peripheral perfusion ● Check wound dressing for staining ● Check any drains for amount and type of drainage ● Observe for any undue restlessness ● Observe for change in responsiveness ● If requested, measure urine volume	8 p.m. 8 a.m. 12 noon until 24 hrs post-op	H.S. 1 Oct.
Pain due to: Surgical wound	Pain controlled to a level acceptable to the patient *Criteria* States that pain is tolerable or not present Able to co-operate comfortably with ALs and nursing activities without distress.	● Observe for signs of discomfort ● Give analgesia as prescribed before pain becomes severe ● Remind patient to ask for analgesia before pain becomes severe ● Help into comfortable position ● If anxiety present, try to reduce by appropriate explanation	8 p.m. 8 a.m. 12 noon until wound is healed	H.S. 6 Oct.

Fig. 4.4   Standard Postoperative Nursing Care Plan

Individual Nursing Care Plan

Name Mrs. Janet Rogers.

Date	Problem and cause(s)	Goal and goal criterion/criteria	Intervention	Dates and initials		
				Evaluate	Item discontinued	Problem resolved
29 Sept.	Use Along With Standard Preoperative Nursing Care Plan					
29 Sept.	Communicating Anxiety about mentally handicapped son's possible reaction to her absence from home and to her hospitalisation	Anxiety allayed criteria. Able to talk easily about son. States that anxiety is less or relieved.	• Give opportunity to talk about son. • Give information about availability of ward telephone. • Speak to patient's sister; encourage her to phone twice daily until son can visit (patient has arranged that he will not visit until day 2 post-op.) • Help patient prepare for son's visit – up in chair, help with appearance.	2 Oct.	HS 29 Sept. HS 29 Sept.	HS 2 Oct.
29 Sept	Eating and Drinking- Overweight Weight 81.2 kg Height 1.626 m	Gradual weight reduction to 63.5 kg (patient's own goal). Criteria Weight will steadily decrease until target reached.	Postpone Implementation until fit postoperatively. • Identify patient's motivation for weight reduction. • Reinforce importance of weight reduction. • Ensure adequate understanding of food constituents. • Suggest that when fit and at home that she records all food and drunk taken for 3 days – and compares with diet sheet.	at 4/52 OP D visit	HS 7 Oct. 7 Oct. 7 Oct. 7 Oct.	
30 Sept.	Use Along With Standard Postoperative Nursing Care Plan					
30 Sept.	Eating and Drinking- Nausea and vomiting due to abdominal surgery.	No nausea or vomiting criteria Able to tolerate controlled intake of oral fluids progressing to full	• Ice only to suck on theatre day • Day 1 post-op, 30 ml orally each hour. • Day 2 post-op, 60 ml orally each hour increasing to full fluids if tolerated. • Give emetics as prescribed.	12 noon 8 pm, 8 am until 3 Oct	HS 30 Sept VM 2 Oct. VM 3 Oct.	HS 3 Oct.

Date	Problem	Goal / Criteria	Nursing action		
	...infection due to high abdominal surgical incision and associated pain, plus smokes 20 cigarettes daily.	criteria No change in patient's normal breathing pattern. No purulent sputum.	...expectoration 5 minutes in every hour while awake. • Ensure adequate pain control. • Help to sit up when in bed. • Start early ambulation as condition allows. • Discourage smoking.	until 4 Oct.	HS 3 Oct.	HS 4 Oct.
2 Oct.	Eliminating- Potential abdominal distension due to post-surgical partial ileus. →	No abdominal distension. criteria "Soft" abdomen + no discomfort.	• Encourage to walk as able. • Record any bowel movement. • Check for start of distension or discomfort; if present, obtain order for suppositories.	12 noon until 3 Oct.	HS 3 Oct.	
3 Oct.	Uncomfortable abdominal distension due to no flatus or faeces passed since surgery.	Relief of abdominal distension and discomfort. criteria "Soft" abdomen. States no discomfort. Flatus or faeces passed.	• Give glycerine suppositories 2. • Do rectal examination; if faeces present, give more suppositories; if bowel empty, pass flatus tube.	HS 3 Oct.	HS 3 Oct.	

Fig. 4.5 Individual Nursing Care Plan

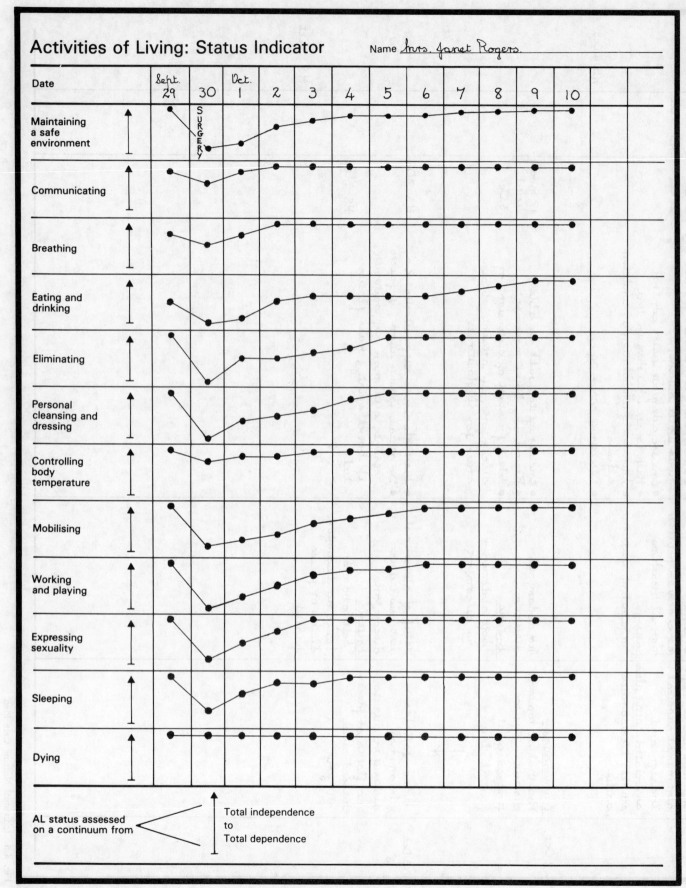

Fig. 4.6 AL Status Indicator

Progress/Evaluation Record

Name *Mrs Janet Rogers.*

Date/time	AL	Evaluation
29 Sept.	Admitted at 1·00pm for elective cholecystectomy	
8 pm.	Communicating.	Not now unduly anxious about surgery. Appears happier about separation from son following evening visit from her sister.
	Eliminating.	Glycerine suppositories 2 given with good result.
	Personal Cleansing and Dressing.	Shave from nipple line to pelvis done.
30 Sept.		
8 am.	Sleeping.	Slept well without sedation.
12·30 pm.	Returned From the Theatre.	Had cholecystectomy; IV infusion in left arm; Nygon drain at wound site.
8 pm.	Breathing.	Normal easy breathing; colour good.
	Eating and Drinking.	Stemetil 12·5 mg. given IM for nausea at 2·50 pm. with good effect; fluids; ice to suck; IV running as charted.
	Eliminating.	No urine passed but no distension or discomfort.
	Mobilising.	Wash, hair combed, teeth brushed at 4·00 pm. Propped up in bed.
	Haemorrhage.	No sign; wound dressing dry.
	Pain.	Omnopon 20 mg. given IM for nausea at 2·50 pm. with good pain relief.
1 Oct.		
8 am.	Eating and Drinking.	Stemetil 12·5 mg. given IM for nausea at 12·30 am. with good effect; sips of water occasionally IV running as charted.
	Eliminating.	No urine passed; slight bladder distension but no discomfort.
	Sleeping.	Slept for short periods.
	Haemorrhage.	No sign.
	Pain.	Omnopon 20 mg. given IM at 12·30 am. with good pain relief.
12 noon	Breathing.	No sign of chest infection Does breathing exercises without being reminded.
	Eating and Drinking.	Vomited small amount. Stemetil 12·5 mg. given IM at 8·30 am. Slight nausea remains but no further vomiting and has tolerated restricted fluids. IV running as charted.

Fig. 4.7 Progress/Evaluation Record

Progress/Evaluation Record

Name Mrs. Janet Rogers

Date/time	AL	Evaluation
	Eliminating.	Passed 200 ml of urine without difficulty at 8·15 am.
	Personal Cleansing and Dressing.	Bedbath given. Wound re-dressed; satisfactory.
	Mobilising.	Up to sit for bedmaking; found this tiring. Pressure areas healthy; moves in bed by herself now. DVT: no signs and doing exercises regularly.
	Haemorrhage.	No sign.
	Pain.	Omnopon 20 mg given I m at 8·30 am with good pain relief.
8 pm.	Eating and Drinking.	Stemetil 12·5 mg given I m at 4·45 pm. with good effect; now tolerating 30 ml of water orally each hour. IV fluids as charted.
	Mobilising.	Felt tired this afternoon; remained in bed.
	Pain.	Omnopon 20 mg given I m at 4·45 pm. with good pain relief.
2 Oct. 8 am.	Eating and Drinking.	No further nausea; tolerating 30 ml of water orally each hour when awake. IV fluids as charted.
	Sleeping.	Slept for most of the night.
	Pain.	No pain until early morning. Omnopon 20 mg given I m at 6·50 am. with good pain relief.
12 noon	Breathing.	No signs of chest infection; doing breathing exercises.
	Eating and Drinking.	No nausea now; tolerating 60-90 ml of water orally each hour. IV fluids as charted.
	Eliminating.	No bowel movement but no discomfort or abdominal distension.
	Personal Cleansing and Dressing.	Bedbath given. Wound drain shortened one inch; drain site satisfactory.
	Mobilising.	Walked round bed and sat in chair for 30 minutes. Pressure areas healthy. DVT: no signs.
	Pain	Omnopon 20 mg given I m at 11·25 am. with good pain relief.

Fig. 4.7 Progress/Evaluation Record (contd)

Progress/Evaluation Record

Name Mrs. Janet Rogers

Date/time	AL	Evaluation
8 pm	Communicating.	Visit from son during afternoon ; reassured about separation.
	Eating and Drinking.	No further nausea ; tolerating free fluid. IV infusion discontinued.
	Mobilising.	Up in chair for 1 hour for visiting ; feels well.
	Pain.	No complaints of pain.
3 Oct.		
8 am.	Sleeping.	Slept well.
	Pain.	No complaints of pain.
12 noon	Breathing	No signs of chest infection.
	Eliminating.	Abdomen distended and patient has some discomfort; no flatus or faeces passed. Glycerine suppositories 2 given at 11·00 am. with no result so far.
	Personal Cleansing and Dressing.	Washed self with some assistance. Wound drain removed ; site satisfactory.
	Mobilising.	Up to sit for most of morning. Walking to toilet with support from nurse. DVT : no signs.
	Pain	DF 118 60 mg orally at 11·55 am.
8 pm.	Eliminating	No result from suppositories ; abdomen remained distended + uncomfortable. Rectal exam. showed empty rectum. Flatus tube passed at 3·00 pm. with good flatus result ; abdomen softer and discomfort relieved.
	Pain	Good control from analgesia previously reported.
4 Oct.		
8 am.	Sleeping.	Sleeping well.
	Pain.	DF 118 60mg given orally at 10 pm. (3 Oct.) with good effect.
12 noon	Breathing.	No signs of chest infection
	Eliminating.	Good bowel movement ; abdomen soft + no discomfort.
	Personal Cleansing and Dressing.	Wound re-dressed ; healing well.

Progress/Evaluation Record   Name Mrs. Janet Rogers

Date/time	AL	Evaluation
	mobilising.	Freely mobile and managing well. DVT : no signs.
	Pain.	DF 118 60 mg given orally at 8.20 am. with good effect.
8 pm.	Pain.	DF 118 60 mg given orally at 1.45 pm. with good effect. DF 118 60 mg given orally at 5.40 pm. Appears to have more pain today than yesterday ; probably due to increased mobility.
5 Oct. 8 am	Sleeping. Pain.	Slept well. No analgesia required.
12 noon	Personal cleansing and Dressing. mobilising. Pain.	Drain site re-dressed; healing. DVT : no signs. No pain.
8 pm.	Pain	DF 118 60 mg given orally at 2.30 pm. with good effect.
6 Oct. 8 am.	Sleeping. Pain.	Slept well. No pain.
12 noon	Personal cleansing and Dressing. mobilising. Pain.	Drain site re-dressed ; satisfactory. DVT ; no signs. DF 118 60 mg given orally at 8.10 am. with good effect.
8 pm	Pain.	No pain.
7 Oct 8 am	Sleeping. Pain	Slept well. No pain.
12 noon	Personal cleansing and Dressing. mobilising. Pain.	Wound re-dressed ; healing well. DVT ; no signs. No pain.
8 pm.	Pain.	No pain.

Fig. 4.7   Progress/Evaluation Record (contd)

Progress/Evaluation Record

Name *Mrs. Janet Rogers*

Date/time	AL	Evaluation
<u>8 Oct.</u> 8 am.	Sleeping. Pain.	Slept well. No pain.
12 noon	Personal Cleansing and Dressing. Mobilising. Pain.	Wound re-dressed; healthy and healing well. DVT; no signs. No pain.
8 pm.	Pain.	No pain
<u>9 Oct.</u> 8 am.	Sleeping. Pain.	Slept well. No pain.
12 noon	Personal Cleansing and Dressing. Mobilising. Pain.	Wound re-dressed; satisfactory. DVT; no signs. No pain.
8 pm.	Pain.	No pain.
<u>10 Oct.</u> 8 am.	Sleeping. Pain.	Slept well. No pain.
12 noon	Personal Cleansing and Dressing. <u>Discharged Home.</u>	Wound stitches removed; wound healed.

5
A health visitor's study of a mother and baby
using the model for nursing

Effie P. Alexander

Introduction

When I was invited to contribute the health visiting study to this book, I had no prior knowledge of the Roper, Logan and Tierney model for nursing. However, I had become involved in using the nursing process and it may be of interest to readers if I first describe that involvement.

The nursing process has been described as a quiet revolution and as such seems to have aroused strong reactions in nurses. These range from indifference and antagonism (because 'we have always done it this way anyway') to enthusiasm for a new way of applying nursing skills and demonstrating their effectiveness. Inevitably the introduction of the nursing process began in hospitals but there is now an increasing interest being shown in the community. This is true of many health visitors who are taking up the challenge to improve standards of professional care by every means possible.

INITIATION TO THE NURSING PROCESS

My initiation to the nursing process began two years ago through a colleague who had attended a conference on the subject of evaluation of community nursing. Considerable emphasis had been put on the nursing process and she introduced this knowledge to a number of health visitors at a staff meeting. As a result an Interest Group was started and about eight health visitors began to meet monthly. Our aims were in the long-term to tackle the problem of how to evaluate the health visitor's work, and in the short-term to improve methods of record keeping, in both cases with particular reference to the nursing process. Even at this early stage I felt that the thinking process and documentation would provide an approach to health visiting which would facilitate care and reflect the work of a health visitor more precisely. Perhaps, I thought, this would be one way of answering the recurring question 'but what exactly does a health visitor do?'

The transition from theory to practice was slow and laborious and I was glad of the support and enthusiasm of the Interest Group. We spent some time reading articles and familiarising ourselves with the nursing process and found that there was much that was an integral part of our practice already. However, with respect to setting goals and evaluation, there was little evidence on records that this had taken place. Indeed as we took a critical look at our own records it became evident that they were more of a historical narrative than a working document.

The challenge of looking at the nursing process brings both a threat and a stimulus. The threat comes from the need to take a critical look at present practice and methods and to probe and admit deficiencies. The stimulus comes from discovering a means to improve and use new knowledge appropriately.

IMPLEMENTING THE NURSING PROCESS

After three months' preparatory work we decided to make a start at implementing the nursing process and chose to do this with every new baby notified. This was a particularly appropriate visit with which to begin as it was a first contact and there was a new record for the documentation. The Interest Group continued to meet regularly and reviewed progress after a further three months. At that time problems and advantages were identified, with the latter being in the majority.

Problems. It was definitely more time-consuming. This was especially true with respect to record-keeping, firstly because there was more to write and secondly the organisation of information was different. It required discipline to keep going in order to evaluate progress effectively.

Advantages. Although there was more writing the records were less vague and more effectively demonstrated the nature of health visiting practice. Plans and the rationale for them were stated so that the means of evaluating work was made possible.

These points summarise some of the outcomes I experienced at these early stages, and since then further developments have confirmed the positive aspects of using the nursing process. From a personal standpoint it is refreshing to have the challenge of innovation and for me it came after practising as a health visitor for five years.

The Interest Group has continued to meet regularly. The 'new' babies with whom we started are now over two years old so that we are now looking at our long-term aim to evaluate the health visitor's work. Inevitably the thinking behind the nursing process has come to be applied in all areas of our work and no longer is it a 'new' or 'different' way of doing things. Indeed it is a relevant approach to health visiting.

Health visiting and the nursing process

A RELEVANT APPROACH

The steps of the nursing process provide a good conceptual framework for health visiting. They are logical and entirely appropriate to practice. Health visitors normally anticipate contact with an individual or family over months or years and actual visits may be separated by weeks or months. To avoid these being unco-ordinated and to provide for continuity of care it is vital that there is assessment, planning and evaluation and that the cycle is continuous.

Memory is fallible and as I, in common with other health visitors, have a caseload number of hundreds it would be impossible to give individualised care without some means of recall. The recording of prospective data helps me to follow up families and do return visits with greater confidence and purpose. Obviously, also, when one health visitor's caseload is passed on to another (for example, if she moves or gives up work) the recorded data is invaluable.

ASSESSMENT

I feel that the skills of assessment are in operation in health visiting combining observational and interviewing techniques to produce a realistic profile of the individual or family situation. Contact may be initiated by the health visitor in the absence of an identified problem or crisis, in this case there will be general aims in view. These are the promotion of health and the prevention of accident and disease. This applies to visiting children under five. Further assessment is specific to the child, but is made in relation to the family and community in which he lives. Thus rates of growth and development, behaviour and progress are seen in context. Factors such as family, housing, finances, culture and class all contribute towards making an accurate assessment, which is essential when there may be differing or conflicting interests to consider.

Assessment may also be in response to a referral from another statutory or voluntary agency, following a patient's discharge from hospital or in response to an individual's request. By carrying out assessment I am helped to understand the situation, to identify needs or problems and to decide whether or not I have any role to play. This helps me to rationalise continuing the contact, referring to another agency or withdrawing.

Assessment involves the investment of time in gathering information by interviewing and observing. But, if done thoroughly, it provides a basis for planned and relevant care. Ultimately time is saved and more achieved when goals and plans relate to reality.

PLANNING

The bridge between assessment and planning is the statement or identification of the goal and as far as general goals are concerned I have plans which are applicable to all children under five. These encompass normal health visiting activities in health education, developmental screening and anticipatory guidance and span the five year period. For example introducing discussion about dental health and home safety, providing literature and encouraging action at appropriate times to enhance the parent's own provision for the child.

As a result of assessment, specific problems or needs are identified, goals set and plans made. In the case of a child I always have to consider the mother for she is usually the person who is acting on the child's behalf. This adds yet another dimension to the situation and can be a complicating factor. If, for example, a baby has a nappy rash then the mother and I agree on the goal which is that the baby will have an intact, healthy skin. However, while the mother thinks that teething has caused the rash, my assessment is that inadequate hygiene is the real cause. Unless I can convince the mother of this, without causing resentment, she will not see the need to implement the plans which will lead to the goal being achieved. My plans will focus on attention to skin and nappy hygiene, whereas the mother may want another cream to apply. This simple example demonstrates the need to deal with the dilemma which arises when a problem is perceived differently by the mother and the health visitor.

In visiting families there may be conflicting needs to consider. For example, the baby is light for dates and needs frequent feeding; the mother has had a Caesarean section and requires rest; the two-year-old is jealous and lively and needs extra attention and play stimulation; and the father's work involves long hours. This demonstrates the complexity which can arise when setting goals and the need for realism in making plans. A list of unworkable plans will only lead to frustration and compound the problem.

The time-scale involved with respect to health visiting is very variable and because contact with a family is not confined to a limited period, as is the case with the majority of hospital admissions, there is more flexibility. This partly compensates for the need to deal with competing interests.

IMPLEMENTATION

In most instances action is taken by the individual themselves or by a relative and this is an important difference between health visiting and the rest of nursing. My role is to motivate a person to take those measures which will enhance their health, and for them to do this in my absence. This is likely to happen only if my assessment of their attitude to a problem has been as accurate as that of the problem itself.

There are many parents who complain about a child's poor sleeping pattern and that they have to take the child into bed with them every night. However I may find that such parents have no intention or inclination to 'do' anything about it themselves. All my advice and plans for the child are rendered nil because the parents are not prepared to implement them and I am not the appropriate person to do it. Through following the steps of the nursing process I have found this area of difficulty considerably resolved and could justify saying 'no action taken'. This helps to avoid the trap of thinking that doing anything is better than doing nothing.

Many nurses are so used to the concept of acting on another's behalf that they find it difficult to relinquish this measure of control. In fact it can be easier to do something yourself than to encourage others to act for themselves. However, if health visitors are to be successful facilitators, they must be prepared to provide the tools for others to use.

EVALUATION

Through the discipline of following the steps of the nursing process it has become much clearer to me how to evaluate my work. Also to demonstrate the benefits or otherwise of various health visiting methods and activities. This discrimination definitely leads to improved practice.

How would I evaluate? To return to the example of the baby with the nappy rash my evaluation would begin before I left the house on the first visit. By getting feedback from the mother to find out how she perceived the problem now and what she was going to do I would establish what she had understood, apart from what she had heard. This is crucial as she is the one who will implement the plan. On a subsequent visit my observation of the baby's skin, combined with what the mother tells me, enables me to assess two things: first, whether or not the baby's skin has healed and, second, what measures the mother actually took. Only then can I evaluate whether or not anything I did or said affected the outcome.

Evaluation is a salutary exercise which prevents me reaching wrong conclusions. There is also a dilemma in some situations where I can only assume that a goal is achieved through my intervention. For example, in one instance I may succeed in encouraging parents to provide a fireguard to prevent the toddler falling in the fire whereas in another I may fail. If neither child is ever burned, can I take credit for the first instance when the second seems to contradict this premise? This is one of the challenges in entering the preventive field.

Applying the model for nursing to health visiting

INITIAL REACTION

My initial reaction to being asked to apply the Roper, Logan and Tierney model for nursing to a health visiting situation was guarded. Their model seemed to me to be orientated to the hospital setting and to patients during illness. This means that the time-scale is usually circumscribed and the nursing work and documentation related to one episode in an individual's life. The focus of planning is on the problems arising from the illness and a discharge point is anticipated. As a health visitor I expect a minimum of five years' contact with a family and view this from the standpoint of 'normality' as opposed to crisis-intervention.

Also it is not only an individual — a new baby — that is involved in health visiting, but a family. Their own home is the context and the intervention involves the offer of a preventive/supportive service rather than nursing care during an episode of illness. So to begin with I could not envisage the model for nursing being relevant to health visiting with children under five, although it did seem a useful framework for nursing in general.

The Patient Assessment Form — based on the model — which we were asked to use at first sight seemed inadequate, both for the type of information required at the initial contact with a mother and new baby, and for other categories of information required to be included subsequently. In the case of a child under five I wish to record information about the birth, the family and the general practitioner at the time of the first contact. Thereafter at appropriate times other essential information should be added, for example, immunisations, hearing test result and entry to any observation register. No place is provided on the form for such information. Also I doubted that one standard form could be used even for the different areas of health visiting work — visits to children, involvement with the handicapped and assessment/support of the elderly.

Activities of living (ALs). To begin with I wondered about the use of ALs in health visiting because the assessment of a baby is made with particular reference to the mother and then the family. The ALs did not seem to allow scope for this as they are assessed in relation to an individual and his/her usual routines. I had been used in assessment to categorising in relation to a group of topics: for example feeding; immunisations; hygiene; first examination of the baby; mother/baby relationship; and mother's health. Fitting these topics into the ALs specified seemed unworkable as I felt that some of my customary topics would span more than one AL thus making the documentation cumbersome. An example of this is given on page 56 where I describe my documentation of the Assessment of Activities of Living.

Actual/potential problems. Reflecting the model's problem-orientated approach, it is intended that problems identified are written on to the Patient Assessment Form, and a distinction made between actual and potential problems. I thought that actual problems would be fairly easy to identify, but immediately felt that potential problems were so numerous in the context of the mother and new baby that it would be impracticable to document them all. On further consideration I decided that it would be feasible if problems specified on the Patient Assessment Form were limited to precise potential problems identified as a result of assessment, rather than the general potential problems which could be envisaged for any child under five. Thus a pre-term baby who has been in the Special Care Unit for two months would have potential sleeping problems, whereas any baby has a potential sleeping problem given certain circumstances which may arise, including teething, illness, colic or overcrowding.

Obviously the new baby's normal condition is one of total dependence so that usual routines sometimes refer to what the mother is doing and sometimes to the behaviour of the baby. The baby may sleep a lot during the day and be wakeful during the night: this is not a problem to the baby but probably it is to the mother who will try to do something about it. It could be argued that this is neither a nurse nor a patient (baby) perceived problem. However it could be a potential problem in that a tired mother is less able to cope satisfactorily. The goal would be an acceptable sleeping routine for the baby, 'acceptable' referring as much to the family as the baby.

Expected outcomes. The points mentioned already regarding setting goals in the nursing process (p. 53) also apply to the model for nursing under discussion. However, there are general aims which involve advice and education, anticipatory guidance and counselling which cannot be fitted easily into this model for nursing. These aspects of health visiting relate closely to the preventive emphasis of family care and are not necessarily dealing with problems which have to be resolved — rather with anticipated needs.

Planning, implementation and evaluation. Here my main reaction related to timing. The model for nursing seems to be considering a situation on a day-to-day basis whereas the health visitor is anticipating long-term contact. During that time planning takes place as a result of assessment and in anticipation of certain stages of the child's development. For example there would be a structured plan to include developmental screening, hearing testing and immunisations. However the underlying principles do apply to health visiting and are vital for continuity of care.

The patient study

INTRODUCTION

For the purpose of this study and the application of the Roper, Logan and Tierney model for nursing in health visiting I selected a family with a new baby. Obviously I could not complete it in the sense of following through for five years, so that for the present exercise I recorded visits until the baby's sixth week and have described plans until three months. As a health visitor I regard this period as crucial to establishing contact with the family and getting a base-line knowledge which guides me in specific planning. The first visit from a health visitor to a new baby is due on the eleventh day after birth and is called the notification visit.

In this case I did not know the family at all so I made a preliminary visit in order to ask for permission to carry out the study. I explained to the mother, Mrs Stewart, that along with several other nurses I was involved in trying out a different approach to nursing and that I would like to do this during my visits for the first few weeks. This would then be written up to become a chapter in a book. I reassured her that no one would have any way of identifying the family and that a different name would be used. Mrs Stewart seemed quite amused by the idea and said that she did not mind at all. I got the impression that she was quite pleased and felt specially selected for the purpose.

THE FIRST VISIT

The actual conduct of the first visit did not vary much from my normal practice. This is due to the structured character of a notification visit and my previous experience in using the nursing process. Prior to the visit I tried to work out what I wanted to discuss regarding each AL, and attempted during the visit to follow them through systematically. From my point of view it was interesting to note that the visit was conducted at a slower pace than is usual for me. I am sure that this was due to the different way my thinking about the visit was organised, and there was more conscious effort in covering all the areas. However this can be seen as a constructive point. It is very easy to adopt a ritualistic approach to particular types of visits and new thinking can prompt useful review.

DOCUMENTING THE ASSESSMENT DATA

Assessment of activities of living. When it came to writing up the visit I was confronted, as always, with a large amount of information which was to be organised and summarised and entered on to the Patient Assessment Form. This took me a long time to think through as some of the routines could have fitted more than one AL. For example the sterilising of bottles is obviously related to the AL of maintaining a safe environment but it is also closely linked to the AL of eating and drinking. Likewise Mrs Stewart's smoking could be relevant to the ALs of maintaining a safe environment and to breathing.

There were two problems identified from assessment of the baby which I could not fit into the ALs — cephalhaematoma and engorged breasts. My 'liaison editor' suggested that cephalhaematoma could be put under medical diagnosis on the Patient Assessment Form and engorged breasts under the AL of expressing sexuality. While I can see the logic of this I am not entirely satisfied with the presentation and feel that cephalhaematoma should be entered with the body of current information about the baby.

On the practical side I found that the space between lines for each AL was too narrow in some cases with the result that writing had to be very small and cramped if all the information obtained had been included. The final presentation is seen in Figure 5.1 (p. 61) and this can be compared with my usual method of writing my records shown in Figure 5.2 (pp. 62-64). The most obvious difference is the layout, and this record is only a plain page, ruled and headed, to provide some structure for reflecting the nursing process.

Patient Assessment Form: biographical and health data. This left-hand side of the form does not have sufficient categories for information. At present there is no standardised child health record for health visiting and in my opinion, most of those in use could be improved, including the one that I am using. Nevertheless they all permit more relevant information to be entered than the Patient Assessment Form being used in this study. The information obtained at the first visit documented on the record I usually use is shown in Figure 5.3 (p. 65) and on the Patient Assessment Form in Figure 5.4 (p. 66). On the latter, two dates are given for date of assessment. I was unable to complete assessment of the ALs until I had actually examined Christine, and as I do not consider it necessary to waken a sleeping baby on my first visit, I had to wait until my second contact to do this. The main omission from this form is the birth history of the baby which would be far more relevant than the bottom section, which is definitely oriented to a crisis situation. The other particular difference between the two forms is that my usual record has space for entering immunisations and hearing test result — it is anticipating routine follow-up of the normal baby. In my view the Patient Assessment Form is more suitable when dealing with an episode of illness.

Planning. In the absence of any particular problem requiring intervention the plans stated are really describing routine health visiting activities in visiting a normal, healthy baby. I feel that this is a framework within which the mother knows what my plan of contact is, and is free herself to contact me at any time. The plans described in this study, shown in Figure 5.5 (p. 67) are simple and predictable and are the first stages in contact which will contribute to the expected outcomes for any child. These are that the child will remain healthy, achieve developmental milestones, complete the immunisation schedule; and avoid accidents. The extent of the health visitor's contribution depends as much on the mother as on the baby. This is one area where the model for nursing seems to be restrictive when applied in practice, there being no scope to develop anything about the mother separate from the 'patient' — the baby. For example I might plan more frequent supervisory visits because a mother shows signs predisposing her to postnatal depression.

Mrs Stewart and I agreed that she would go to the local child health clinic when she wanted Christine weighed and for immunisations, but would come to the group practice's surgery where I run a well baby clinic for developmental screening. The reason for this is that the family live four miles from the surgery and are dependent upon public transport for travel. This is one of the constraints present when planning as a health visitor. I am in regular contact with the health visitors at the local clinic so that it is possible to maintain continuity of care.

During the course of the first six weeks of the baby's life, Mrs Stewart did attend the local clinic and on each occasion the baby's weight gain was satisfactory. My second contact with the family was, as planned, eleven days after the notification visit. In the intervening time I had confirmed the other children's immunisation schedule and the family medical history from the general practitioner notes. This, combined with the discussion which I had had with Mrs Stewart previously, is the procedure followed prior to getting the parents' signature on the immunisation form. This form states that the parent wishes to have the child immunised.

The baby was awake during this second visit so I was able to examine the baby and confirm that she was a normal, healthy baby. The written outline of this examination is included in my report of this visit (Fig. 5.2, p. 63). I noted that both the cephalhaematoma and engorged breasts were beginning to resolve and drew Mrs Stewart's attention to this. She was reassured and relieved.

We discussed the baby's feeding and I discovered that Mrs Stewart had changed the baby milk to another brand 'because she was windy'. Since then the baby had been settled and there was no problem. It is relatively common for mothers to think that a change of milk is the answer to all problems related to feeding. If an improvement follows, then the mother is sure about it. There is no argument possible when this 'evidence' is produced and as a health visitor I can only suggest that any further change would be inadvisable. I do this on the basis that a feeding problem is more likely to be due to the techniques employed being faulty, for example the size of the hole in the teat being too small or large for the baby.

Mrs Stewart then told me that the baby appeared to be contented and was sleeping well between feeds: she was settled in a routine and this was being respected by the rest of the family.

The timing and content of this visit followed the plan described in Figure 5.5 (p. 67) and included evaluation and re-assessment. The evaluation related to the immunisation default, cephalhaematoma, and maternal anxiety and the feeding was re-assessed. The mother and I then decided that she would take the baby to the local clinic in one or two weeks' time and bring her to the surgery well-baby clinic at six weeks for routine developmental screening.

In fact Mrs Stewart telephoned me two weeks later as she was worried about the baby's noisy breathing. The information which she gave me: that the baby could breathe through her nose and that feeding was unaffected helped me to decide to visit rather than refer this call to the general practitioner. On examination I could see that the baby was well hydrated and a good colour. The breathing was quiet and Mrs Stewart said there was no diarrhoea or vomiting. This assessment demonstrated that there was in fact no problem with the baby and that the noise Mrs Stewart was hearing was due to normal nasal secretions. I reassured Mrs Stewart about this and advised her to raise the head of the carry-cot mattress slightly to help drainage of the secretions. Mrs Stewart accepted my explanation and said that she felt reassured. I then outlined what symptoms constitute a problem for the baby so that she would know when to call the general practitioner. While examining the baby I also noted that the engorged breasts had resolved and the cephalhaematoma was almost fully resolved.

Mrs Stewart brought Christine for her routine check on the 5th November. In the group practice where I am based I do the developmental screening and only refer to the doctors when necessary. The baby was assessed on the four areas considered — posture and large movements; vision; hearing and speech; and social behaviour and play — and the baby was within limits of normal in every respect. I described this examination to Mrs Stewart as I was doing it and used it as an opportunity for health education, talking, for example, about the anterior fontanelle, routine skin care and anticipating the next stages in development. The baby's weight was 4.31 kg which combined with her general appearance of well-being indicated that she was thriving.

There had been no further anxiety about the baby's breathing and Mrs Stewart had implemented the suggestion to raise the head of the mattress. The cephalhaematoma was fully resolved. My impression following assessment was of a normal, contented baby with the mother enjoying her and coping well.

Throughout each visit I followed the steps of the nursing process with particular reference to the plan (Fig. 5.5, p. 67).

However, I also allowed the mother the opportunity to bring up any topic of concern or interest to her.

At this stage I arranged to visit the family in one month's time and my main purpose was to discuss immunisations and encourage Mrs Stewart to bring Christine to the clinic when these were due to commence. In the intervening time she would continue to attend the local clinic for routine weighing — in the absence of any concern about either underweight or overweight, this means as often as the mother wants.

DISCUSSION OF ASSESSMENT OF ALs

Although initially I had reservations about the relevance to health visiting of the ALs' focus of the model for nursing, having tried it out I did find that this framework encouraged a comprehensive assessment of the baby. However, as this assessment data will require frequent revision and updating relative to the baby's growth and development and changing needs I have discussed the wider issues which proceed from the gathered facts. Also the assessment is made with the baby as a passive participant in the interview where the mother and I are talking about her and trying to interpret her needs and feelings. Objective observation on my part combined with the mother's subjective information are elements required in assessment of the baby. To illustrate this some comments follow about each of the ALs in turn.

Maintaining a safe environment. This AL does have particular relevance to health visiting. In this study I discovered that bringing diverse topics together because they all related to accident prevention and promotion of safety concentrated my thinking and directed me during the visit. I think that this may also help to heighten the mother's awareness of the need to take active measures in maintaining a safe environment. As the baby progresses towards independence and mobility this assessment will have to be revised regularly. However, this should be in anticipation of what is going to happen in order to plan for prevention. For example, the goal in the area of home safety would be that the child will not have any accidents and planning would be to that end in relation to each child's particular circumstances. Therefore fireguards, stair-gates and plug guards need to be in situ before the baby's first exploration of the dangers which fires, stairs and electricity sockets present.

Communicating. The assessment details gathered present a profile of normality, and later queries about delay or deviation from the normal can then be measured against recorded facts. This is comparable to describing a patient's usual routine and the factors which have disrupted it. I found it interesting to discuss vision, hearing and pre-speech sounds under the heading of communicating, as it encouraged attention to the baby's need to be actively stimulated for these areas to develop. It is important to discover parental attitudes to communicating with their baby. Some parents need to be shown that the baby is in fact responding to a need when he is crying and that the art of communicating here is discovering what each cry means. Also, as in this case, it is necessary to advise against excessive stimulation of the new baby which could make her fretful.

Breathing. The character of breathing is particularly important in this first assessment. During the visit I described my observations of the baby's breathing to the mother and then indicated the different situations which could cause the breathing to change. For example a dry atmosphere or mucous secretions in the nasal passages can cause a baby's breathing to sound noisy. Many parents hearing this for the first time become very alarmed, and I am often asked for advice about it. Provided the baby can still breathe through the nose and feeding is unaffected, parents can be reassured that the baby is well. However, I always advise parents to seek medical advice about any change in the character of a baby's breathing that is unexplained or is worrying them. It was about this type of situation that the mother first 'phoned me — as described on page 57. This is using the assessment as an opportunity for simple education in the hope that parents will be spared unnecessary anxieties but will also take prompt and appropriate action when required. The mother's smoking is relevant to this AL in particular, although it could also be included in the AL of maintaining a safe environment.

Eating and drinking. In making an assessment of this AL, I want to obtain accurate information about the present situation and get some insight into parental practices and attitudes with respect to eating and drinking. This may be one of the areas about which health visitors are most often asked for advice. There is such diversity of opinions about food and nutrition that good assessment is vital in order to advise appropriately. For instance a mother may say that she does not give her baby any solids and in response to further questioning admit that she adds cereal to the bottle. This may be because she perceives 'solids' as being given with a spoon. Similarly a mother can say she gives the child vegetables and the health visitor then discovers that vegetables means tinned beans and spaghetti only. As well as finding out about the baby's intake of food it is necessary to check the preparation of the feeds. A mother may know that she should reconstitute four scoops of milk powder with 120 ml of water. However, sometimes mothers put the milk powder into the bottle and 'top up' with water to the required level, thus reducing the actual volume of fluid. In fact the fluid should be measured separately. It is detail like this that needs to be checked. Also it is important to find out if the mother realises that a baby can be thirsty as well as hungry. Occasionally thirsty babies are given more milk (their food) and so become more thirsty and irritable when all that they require is a drink of cooled boiled water. Other topics will also be included in the assessment of this AL, for example winding, vomiting, feeding techniques, choice of milk powder, timing of feeds and the baby's weight.

Eliminating. When assessing this AL I asked the mother to describe to me the baby's stools and urine and the frequency of elimination. This gives me a profile of the usual routine, and subsequent changes can be measured against this to some extent. However, a normal process of change is anticipated because of the variation in food intake which occurs. Firstly the increasing volume of milk and later the introduction of solids causes changes in the consistency, colour and frequency of stools. Problems which arise in connection with this AL are often 'parent-perceived' problems and are called by them 'diarrhoea' or 'constipation'. These terms are used to indicate frequent or infrequent stools and this indiscriminate use of words leads parents to feel something needs to be done. For example a breast-fed baby may have a bowel movement once every three or four days. If the mother's expectation is a daily bowel movement she concludes that the baby is 'constipated' and proceeds to offer extra water or fruit juice. The baby may then have 'diarrhoea' which is really diet-induced frequency of stools. All this can be a source of great anxiety to parents so that, as in many other aspects of health visiting, anticipatory guidance should be given. Discussion of this AL with the mother is very closely linked with that of eating and drinking, and personal cleansing and dressing, as dietary habits and skin hygiene are the mother's responsibility entirely at this stage. What she does affects this routine directly, and one of the possible consequences of it — nappy rash.

Personal cleansing and dressing. In assessing this AL, I am looking for a suitable, effective routine which promotes skin care and causes the baby to feel comfortable. Mothers may have great variations in their approach to this routine; for example a baby may be bathed in the morning or the evening, every day or each alternate day. The detail of when it is done is interesting; however, the important observation is the effect of whatever action is being taken. Routine examination of the naked baby gives the health visitor the ideal opportunity to see the results of skin care and to educate the mother where necessary. For example, some babies present with a patch or cradle cap over the anterior fontanelle because the mother is nervous of touching it. Many babies have intermittent or transient skin rashes which may be due to heat or irritation from clothing. Reassurance, accurate information and advice about such matters should promote the mother's confidence and increase her enjoyment of this routine.

My normal practice is to ask if the baby's nappy area is cleansed at every nappy change. From experience I have found that if the baby has only passed urine and the skin does not look 'dirty' some mothers just put more cream on and then a fresh nappy. This is one occasion when I would actually demonstrate the point using cotton wool so that the mother could see the colour of the urine on it. This has more effect than mere words. Associated with the assessment of this AL is the washing of clothes and nappies, suitability of clothing and the array of soaps, powders, lotions and creams which confront a mother. Basic and thorough hygiene is the most effective means of skin care — soap, water and a towel are usually all that is required. The rest provide the frills and pleasant smells of this care.

Controlling body temperature. The young baby is particularly susceptible to variations of body temperature. The actual appearance and feel of the baby's skin will assist in monitoring this and is the starting point of assessment. Then the other factors affecting the baby's temperature need to be assessed. These are room temperature, clothing and bedding and the weather, when the baby is outside. There are so many variables that it would be difficult to anticipate them all with the mother. I usually demonstrate with the baby what is normal and then advise the mother to adjust the other factors appropriately if the baby seems to be too hot or too cold. In this instance the room was very warm and I did suggest that the mother remove two of the four covers which were on the baby. I could anticipate discussing financial matters in relation to this AL as fear of high bills are a considerable constraint on providing adequate heating.

Mobilising. Having ascertained that the baby's locomotor development is within normal limits, assessment of this AL focuses on environmental and social factors. These include the scope given to the baby to move freely and the manner in which she is handled. In the course of my second visit I noticed that the mother handled the baby confidently and expertly. Although this is her third child I would not assume that this would be the case as it was six years since the previous child was born. A mother can be tense, nervous or relaxed when handling a baby and this has an affect on the response of a baby who reacts to the mother. As the baby develops independent mobility I think that I would link this AL closely to maintaining a safe environment as indicated in the discussion of that AL (p. 57).

Working and playing. I found it difficult to know if there was anything to assess about the baby in relation to this AL. However, the nursing activities described under 'implementation' on the summary chart at the end of Chapter 15 in *The Elements of Nursing* including 'preventing boredom' and 'providing stimulation', are relevant to a baby's needs even from the first few weeks. This obviously connects with the AL of communicating, and can focus on what the mother and family do to interest the baby and encourage him to respond and to enjoy play. Some parents need help and guidance to overcome the embarrassment they feel when talking to a baby who cannot talk back and to see the point of 'playing' with the baby. The baby's own response is ultimately the greatest encouragement and reason for doing it.

Expressing sexuality. As with the previous AL, I thought that I would have nothing to assess concerning the baby. Indirect evidence that the sex of a baby is very important to the parents may be concluded from the fact that this is the first information they are given at the birth followed swiftly by a comment on the baby's condition. Attitude to the baby's sex could have a bearing on the quality of care given and the amount of attention given by one or other of the parents. For example, if a father wants a boy 'to carry on the name' he might have difficulty in reconciling himself to his third daughter. In some ethnic or cultural groups the sex of the baby will have different connotations, and as a health visitor I have to take account of this when giving advice. For the purpose of this study I did include engorged breasts in the assessment of this AL as suggested. As there is already a boy and girl in this family the mother said that they had had no preference regarding the baby's sex.

Sleeping. In assessing this AL, I normally find out where, when and how the baby sleeps. It is always essential to find out the mother's perception of how long the baby sleeps. Most people find broken nights and disturbed sleep difficult to cope with and a baby's night wakefulness can be exaggerated because of the way a mother is feeling. Assessment must take account of this as this is one area where there can be competing interests. Advice often tends towards compromise as the baby is gradually integrated into the family, and they both adjust to one another. The baby's need for sleep changes markedly during the first year of life, and while encouraging a regular routine the health visitor often has to remind the mother to take account of these changes. The sleeping pattern described for the baby in the study is entirely normal and requires no comment. It is recorded for purposes of comparison.

Dying. In the study there was nothing to record in the assessment of this AL. However, I can think of some situations where this would be raised by a mother or family. For example, if there has been a stillbirth or infant death previously, there is considerable anxiety about any baby born subsequently. There can also be fears of a cot death. These fears are very real to those experiencing them. If a baby is pre-term and has problems during and after birth requiring intensive or special care the parents are confronted with the possibility of the baby dying. They need considerable support while the baby is kept in hospital and after discharge. Hospitalisation of a baby for any reason is a traumatic experience for parents and the separation of mother and baby can feel like a death. It has been known for mothers who have to leave their babies in the Special Care Unit and go home — perhaps because there are other children to attend to — to wonder if they really have had a baby. It is like a bereavement. The health visitor would have a supportive role in this type of situation.

Reflections and conclusions

Well what do I feel has come out of this study — for me personally and for health visiting? The project in general was a challenge to me to look at methods of work and the rationale for them, and I enjoyed the stimulus of thinking through familiar situations from a different standpoint. The real struggle came at the writing-up stage of the project and the difficulty was mainly due to the fact that the time allotted for the family contact (six weeks) was too short. The pace of health visiting is slower than that of acute nursing, and to give a true profile of the baby I felt that I had to include current and prospective details relating to prevention of disease and accident as well as the promotion of health.

I was already thoroughly convinced of the relevance of the nursing process to health visiting and thus found that adopting ALs as the framework for assessment was the greatest innovation for me regarding the project. I like the emphasis which this places on looking at the individual as a whole person rather than a collection of body-systems. This is an advantage to health visiting where the individual is seen as a whole and then by the assessment, particular problems or needs are identified. The disadvantage with the baby is that definite changes take place quickly and the initial assessment is soon out of date. However, it remains relevant as an important baseline.

I have already described my initial reaction to the Roper, Logan and Tierney model for nursing on page 54. Having tested it out in the project — which was a classic health visiting situation — I have modified my attitude. The thinking steps employed are entirely appropriate to health visiting. The application described in *Learning to Use the Process of Nursing* is to a selected group — those in need of nursing because they have a health problem — and this is different from health visiting where the selected group may include everyone in an age group irrespective of their having a health problem or not. However, the nursing concern 'with helping people at all stages of their life span to achieve their optimal level of health' (*The Elements of Nursing*, p. 61) is common to every nursing discipline. Therefore it may be possible to have one model for nursing encompassing them all. In my opinion the Roper, Logan and Tierney model for nursing usefully demonstrates this possibility. Apart from the need for more appropriate forms for documentation, and the fact that my project is really unfinished until the child is five, I found this model working for me as I applied it to the situation.

I can envisage applying this model for nursing in other health visiting situations. For example when visiting the elderly or handicapped, assessment of ALs is particularly apposite. Each one allows for a consideration of the interrelation between physical, psychological and social factors which affect the individual's ability to cope. This comprehensive method of assessment should facilitate planning which will be relevant both to the individual and the family/community in which he/she lives.

I see evaluation as the key to improving the quality of nursing and the nursing process as the means employed. Evaluation provides the measure by which we can judge our effectiveness and competence, and the planned activity of the nursing process provides a methodical approach to increasing both. This should mean that the individual receives a better quality of care and the nurse will have increased job satisfaction. That would be my goal for health visiting.

Assessment of Activities of Living

Date 12 Oct.

AL	Usual routines: what he/she can and cannot do independently	Patient's problems (actual/potential) (p)= potential
● Maintaining a safe environment	Bottles/teats sterilized correctly by chemical method. Parents wish baby to be immunised though sibs. schedule unsatisfactory. Fireguard round coal fire normally in situ. but as family pet–cat net on carry cot.	● (P) Immunisation default.
● Communicating	Normal cry. Startles to sudden sounds. Turns towards light. Extended family visit frequently and likes to "play" with Christine – always picking her up.	● (P) Over-stimulation/ disturbed routine
● Breathing	Quiet regular nose breathing. Skin colour pink. Mother smokes 20 per day – not inclined to stop.	● (P) Smoke inhalation
● Eating and drinking	Bottle fed. Ostermilk complete formula: 120 mls. approx. 4 hrly. Reconstituted correctly. Sucks well. No vomiting. Cooled boiled water given as a drink when necessary. Intake satisfactory in relation to age, birth weight and gestation.	
● Eliminating	Soft yellow stools – 2 or 3 in 24 hours. Passes urine regularly.	
● Personal cleansing and dressing	Thick hair – shampooed daily. Bathed daily in the morning. Napkin area washed at each change. Skin hygiene satisfactory. Towelling nappies used. Zinc castor Oil ointment applied to skin. Dressed appropriately.	
● Controlling body temperature	Clothing and bedding satisfactory. Living room heated with coal fire – atmosphere very warm. In parents bedroom at night – heated 2 hours before. Mother aware of need to monitor clothes and environment. Skin feels dry and warm.	
● Mobilising	Normal posture and muscle tone. Primitive reflexes present. Kicks vigorously when changed or bathed. Mother handles baby confidently	
● Working and playing	Mother and rest of family speak to and play with baby when awake.	
● Expressing sexuality	Engorged breasts.	● (P) maternal anxiety ● (P) Infection
● Sleeping	Sleeps well between feeds. Wakens when hungry. Wakeful period: 1800 – 2100. Sleeps in carry cot at present.	
● Dying		

Fig. 5.1 Patient Assessment Form: assessment of ALs (first assessment of baby)

Date of Visit	Source	Topic/Problem	Assessment/Evaluation	Aims Plans next contact. H.V.'s initials E. P. Alexander
1 Oct.	V	Notification Visit	Hospital and midwife's discharge satisfactory.	
		Baby	Sleeping at time of visit – not examined. Mother (M) reports baby well and contented. In carry-cot in living room – heated with coal fire. Fireguard in situ.	Routine surveillance and health care
		Feeding	Bottle fed on Ostermilk complete formula 120 mls. approximately 4 hrly. Feeds well, no vomiting. Stools soft, yellow, regular. Correct reconstitution of milk powder.	
			Milton method of sterilisation of bottles/teats.	Plan.
			Cooled boiled water given periodically as a drink.	I 1st examination of baby
		① Cephalhaematoma	① side M anxious – has been told resolution will occur. Reassured	II monitor ①②
		② Engorged Breasts	M reports no redness but is anxious. Informed no action necessary – will resolve.	
		Immunisations	M uncertain of siblings' schedule. No significant family medical history reported. No contra-indications from baby's history. Parents wish baby immunised.	III H.N. to check sibs. immunisation schedule. Consent form to be signed.
		Clinic	Will attend local clinic for routine weighing. To surgery for developmental checks.	IV Routine support
		Maternal Health	Cervical tear: PPH required 3 units packed cells. Hb. 10.3 taking Fe Sulphate 200 mg T.I.D. 6th. day: superficial venous thrombosis R. leg	

Fig. 5.2 Usual method of documenting assessment data

Date of Visit	Source	Topic/Problem	Assessment/Evaluation	Aims Plans next contact H.V.'s initials E.P. Alexander
			Rx Butazolidine 100mg T.I.D-resolved. Reports feeling well, not unduly tired and coping with baby. Smokes 20/day: not inclined to stop. Advised against smoking near baby.	☑ Mr to contact H.N. if any problem.
		Family Planning Post natal	To G.P for post natal check and will re-commence oral contraceptive pill.	
		Father	Shift work as a miner. On holiday just now. Gives Mr. help in the home - Mr. says taking more interest in this baby than he did with siblings.	
		Family	All interested in baby - many visitors all wanting to see and hold her.	Local clinic 1 wk. Home visit 2 wks.
		Housing.	Only 2 bedrooms - will need to consider a move, but wish coal fire as fuel subsidised.	
8 Oct.	Local clinic		Wt. 8.5½ Baby windy.	
12 Oct.	V	Immunisations	Both sibs D.T.P and Polio x 3 - schedule unsatisfactory due to defaulting. Consent form signed.	
		First Examination	Anterior fontanelle 2f.b. Eyes ✓ mouth ✓ skin ✓ Umbilicus ✓ Reflexes ✓ muscle tone ✓ Posture ✓ Turns to light and responds to loud noises.	To surgery 5 Nov.
		① Cephalhaematoma ② Engorged Breasts	Both resolving.	for 6 week check.

Date of Visit	Source	Topic/Problem	Assessment/Evaluation	Aims Plans next contact H.V.'s initials E. P. Alexander
		Feeding	M changed to S M A gold cap "because baby windy."	
			Feeding well 120 mls 4 hrly : now reported settled.	
			Advised no further change in milk formula.	
26 Oct.	V	③ Noisy Breathing	plus occasional cough. Feeding well, no diarrhoea	
	M's request		or vomiting. Baby breathing quietly. M anxious.	
			Reassured noise due to nasal secretions : advised to	
			raise head of mattress slightly. Informed what signs	I M will contact
			would indicate a problem requiring medical aid.	G.P. if baby unwell.
26 Oct.	V	① ②	① Almost fully resolved ② Resolved	
29 Oct.	Local clinic		Wt. 9·1	
5 Nov.	Surgery	Six Weeks	Normal posture and muscle tone. Pull to sit — some	
			head lag. Prone lifts head. Ventral suspension ✓	Home visit 1 month
			Reflexes normal	I Immunisations
			Focusing and following.	II Anticipate
			Responds to sounds. Quietens when spoken to. M	weaning.
			reports vocalising.	
			Smiles responsively. Alert, lively baby.	Take leaflets
			Wt. 9·8 Thriving, contented baby.	
		①	Resolved.	

Fig. 5.2 Usual method of documenting assessment data (contd)

REG. No................... WARD C.H.11

AT RISK   Yes/(No) | Give Dates of:-
HANDICAPPED   Yes/(No) | Triple and Polio (1) ....
PHENYLK. TEST   +ve/(-ve) | Vaccinations   (2)........
HEARING TESTING......... | (3)........
Result .... | Measles Vacc. (1) ....
                                             | Smallpox Vacc. (1) ....
FIREGUARD   (Yes)/No | B.C.G.   (1) ....
                 On loan/owned | Boost Dip. Tet.
                                             | and Polio   (1) ....
                                             | Others   ....

COMMUNITY HEALTH SERVICE
CHILD HEALTH SERVICE

HEALTH VISITOR'S HOME VISITING RECORD

CHILD

                    or Owens
Surname... Stewart..............Address   (1) 45/3 Jane St............... Flat middle

Christian Names. Christine...........   (2)..................................

Date of Birth 20/9.......M.(F)/Leg./Illeg. (3)..................................

Where born St. marys maternity Hospital   (4)..................................

Birth Weight 3.69 kg.   (5)..................................

Gestation 41 weeks...............   (6)..................................

                                                                    'Ph. 996 6501

Religion R/C....... Reference Address mrs. mary Owens 10/2 Jane Street...........

Abnormalities present..

Family Doctor (1) Dr. Brown..........   Address (1) 6 Fort Gardens............

            (2).....................   (2)..............................

            (3).....................   (3)..............................

School....................... H.V. prior to School Entry........................

CUT HERE —

MOTHER
                                                          31/3
                                                              co-habiting
Full Name.... Janet (Owens)............... Age 27...M./S./W./Separated
                                            ① Sarah age 9
                                              David age 7

No. of Previous Pregnancies. 2.......... { Born Alive 2................ Stillborn ....

                                          { Died...................... Miscarriages...........

Health:
During Pregnancy good...

Labour:
Duration and Character S.N.D..

FATHER

Full Name... Charles Stewart... 31 years..
Occupation.. miner...

Fig. 5.3 Usual method of documenting biographical and health data

Patient Assessment Form

Date of admission (*first visit*) 1 October   Date of assessment 1 October

Surname *Stewart or Owens*   Forenames *Christine*

Male ☐   Age ☐   ✓ Single/Married/Widowed   Prefers to be addressed as
Female ✓   Other

Date of birth *20 September*

Address of usual residence   *45/3 Jane Street*

Type of accommodation *Council flat : middle in block of six. 2 bedrooms.*

Family/Others at this residence *Parents ; 1 brother and 1 sister*

Next of kin   Name *Alan Stewart*   Address *as above*

Relationship *Father*   Tel. no. *996 6501*

Significant others   Relatives/Dependents

Helpers

Visitors

Occupation   *Father : coal miner*

Religious beliefs and relevant practices *Roman Catholic*

Patient's perception of current health status

Reason for admission/referral *Routine health visiting follow-up of new baby*

Medical diagnosis   *Cephalhaematoma*

Past medical history

Allergies *none*   Significant life crises

Fig. 5.4 Patient Assessment Form: biographical and health data

Problems with ALs.

AL	Problem	Goal	Health Visiting Intervention	Evaluation
• maintaining a safe environment.	(P) Immunisation default.	Completed schedule.	Obtain informed consent. Home visit prior to starting.	15-18 months.
• Communicating.	(P) Over-stimulation.	Contented baby.	Encourage routine to meet baby's needs.	Each visit.
• Breathing.	(P) Smoke inhalation.		Inform parents of risks. Advise no smoking near baby.	Each visit.
• Expressing Sexuality.	maternal anxiety/ (P) Infection. re baby's engorged breasts	Decreased anxiety. No infection.	Reassure resolution normal. Advise no interference. G.P. if inflamed or painful.	Within 2 weeks.

Other Problems.

Cephalhaematoma.	(P) Trauma. maternal anxiety.	Intact skin. Decreased anxiety.	Advise extra care. Reassure resolution normal.	Weeks to months.

Other Topics.

Feeding.
Goal: Appropriate food and drink intake. Normal growth.
Plan: Reassess and advise when necessary / Each visit.
Anticipate weaning, discuss and give leaflets 2½ - 3 months.
Weight checks at local well baby clinic.

Health Visitor.
Goal: Family understand role and use service appropriately
Plan: Describe what health visitor does and explain purpose of visits.
Encourage contact for advice and support.

Planned contact.
Home visit at 3 weeks - routine follow up of notification visit.
Surgery at 6 weeks - developmental screening.
Home visit at 10 weeks - discuss commencing of immunisations.
anticipate weaning - take leaflets.
Clinic at 3 months - commence immunisations.
Periodic attendance at local clinic for weight checks.

Fig. 5.5 Health visiting plan

6
A midwife's study of a mother and baby

using the model for nursing

Euphemia M. Taylor and Molly Coventry

Introduction

REASON FOR PARTICIPATION

A phone call, followed by a letter from Churchill Livingstone inviting us to participate in the application of this model for nursing to midwifery was the main reason for our involvement in this project. Since we already had a considerable interest in the nursing process, having read articles in the nursing journals, it seemed a good opportunity to put into practice what had, until now, been theoretical knowledge. Another reason influencing our decision was the challenge of tackling a new project.

THE HOSPITAL

This modern maternity hospital with 100 beds and 25 special care cots is situated in pleasant surroundings in the suburbs of a large city. The prenatal and postnatal areas are on the same floor comprising four-bedded units, single rooms and a patients' sitting room. All rooms have their own toilet, bidet and shower facilities en suite. There are two isolation rooms in each ward which have their own small nursery adjacent. In the labour unit there are nine delivery rooms which are adjacent to the admission suite and operating theatre.

THE CONTRIBUTORS

A midwifery clinical teacher was selected to work on the project with a student midwife, and a Director of Nurse Education collaborated with them. But since the clinical teacher had responsibility for teaching in the whole department, it was difficult to maintain continuity in relation to one ward and one patient; however, we were fortunate and

had the full co-operation of the ward sister throughout the project. The student midwife to be selected required to have some previous knowledge and experience of postnatal care, and there was only one student midwife, newly allocated to the unit, who met the criteria for participation in the project.

SELECTION OF THE PATIENT

The intention was to select a primigravid patient, after a normal delivery, who wished to breast feed her baby, but on the set day, only one patient out of the five admitted was having her first baby. Following induction of labour and a normal delivery of a live baby girl, this patient was selected, although she wished to bottle feed her baby. After explanation of the model for nursing, Mrs Temple willingly agreed to take part in the project, knowing that later this would be incorporated in a chapter of a book.

Prior knowledge of the nursing process/model for nursing

As a clinical teacher I had previously read a number of care studies incorporating the nursing process and problem solving care plans which had been published in the nursing journals. The student midwife had no practical experience of the nursing process although she understood the basic concepts. The time factor in coming to grips with the particular approach of the model for nursing was considerable, both for teacher and student.

Trial runs in applying the model for nursing

In view of the unfamiliarity of the assessment form and the initial difficulty of thinking in terms of ALs, it was decided to have a preliminary try-out of the assessment form, and a student midwife who had previous experience of a type of nursing process was asked to participate. She quickly grasped the principles and the approach of the model for nursing and did not encounter any real difficulties. While completing the assessment form, the student elicited information regarding social problems which were making the patient 'anxious'. It is interesting to note that no other member of staff was aware of these problems and it helped the staff in their approach to the patient, who appeared on the surface to be happy and contented with no obvious problems. The student herself commented on the beneficial aspects of the total approach of the assessment form and the complete picture it gave of the patient.

A second student midwife, indeed the one who was selected for the main project, also carried out a preliminary trial using the Patient Assessment Form. She too was unfamiliar with the assessment form, so it was imperative that she had time to absorb the salient points in the model for nursing. After a suitable period, the clinical teacher and this student midwife together completed an assessment of a patient who was happy to co-operate; a separate assessment was carried out on the baby. This was a useful exercise for the student which gave her more confidence in approaching the actual project in which Mrs Temple was the selected mother.

Application of the model for nursing

When Mrs Temple returned to the ward from the labour suite she was allocated a single room to provide privacy for completion of the Patient Assessment Form (Figs 6.1, 6.2 pp. 72-74). On her third postnatal day she was transferred to a four-bedded unit. The factors which emerged from the assessment were:

● the pregnancy was unplanned
● Mrs Temple's home was small and had an outside toilet
● her husband was unemployed
● she intended to return to work after maternity leave.

This information was useful, enabling staff to ensure that Mrs Temple was given guidance about attendance at a family planning clinic, especially in view of her husband's inability to obtain employment. Similarly it was important to find out what provision there was for bathing and so on in relation to the outside toilet.

ACTUAL AND POTENTIAL PROBLEMS

The first actual problem was the difficulty Mrs Temple found in bottle feeding her baby. She was very tense, held the baby awkwardly and was very tentative about the whole procedure. The student carried out demonstration feeds on more than one occasion and then watched Mrs Temple feeding baby Laura. After three days she was much more confident and relaxed while feeding her baby.

Another actual problem was slight intermittent abdominal pain which Mrs Temple complained of on her second postnatal day. The student reported this to sister and observations of TPR, urinary output and lochial discharge were carried out, but these were all normal and the abdominal pain settled after one day.

A potential problem was infection, so Mrs Temple was given advice on vulval toilet, use of the bidet and shower and the importance of hand washing. She did not develop any infection during the postnatal period.

On the third postnatal day it was observed that involution of the uterus was static. When questioned, Mrs Temple indicated that she had not had a bowel movement since the birth of her baby. Two suppositories were prescribed and the result was satisfactory. On checking Mrs Temple's fundal height, it had decreased by 2.5 cm. She was also given advice about taking more roughage in her diet and thereafter constipation ceased to be a problem.

Other problems for Mrs Temple were lack of knowledge about family planning and making up artificial feeds for her baby, as well as apprehension about bathing the baby. These were resolved as indicated in Figure 6.3 (p. 75).

At two days old the baby presented a problem when she developed red buttocks (Fig. 6.4, p. 77). Mrs Temple was instructed to wash the napkin area thoroughly and pat it dry, then to apply white vaseline. After 24 hours the redness disappeared and there was no recurrence. Daily examination of the baby was carried out regarding possible sites of infection but she remained healthy and free from infection. Baby Laura had no respiratory difficulty at birth or during the remainder of the postnatal period. Similarly jaundice was not evident during the first week after birth.

NURSING PLAN

It became clear that in addition to the assessment form, another type of nursing plan would be necessary for the routine care of mother and baby. Such a plan for the mother was devised using the ALs as headings (Fig. 6.5, p. 78) but much more time would be needed to plan and implement it, trying it out over several months and making the necessary adjustments. Because of the time constraint it was not possible during this project, to put it into effect. A similar nursing plan for the baby was not produced, because of the need to think through the different aspects, and time again was the enemy.

As well as a temperature and blood pressure chart, a further chart is required at the bed-side indicating the daily nursing needed by mother and baby, with spaces for recording signatures to confirm that the planned interventions have been carried out.

Advantages of the model for nursing

By using the assessment form, a total picture of the patient emerged, enabling the nurse to plan more effective nursing interventions. The plan also highlighted actual and potential problems, alerting the student to plan effective measures to deal with them. The fact that one student was responsible for one patient over several days led to excellent communication. The rapport between student and patient was such that not only was the patient co-operative, but felt free to ask the student various questions and to voice her concerns. The student became aware of Mrs Temple's apprehension in caring for her baby and was able to give her the kind of help and support which she needed to achieve satisfactory bonding. The end result of all this for the patient was a sense of satisfaction, feeling that her difficulties, however slight, had been overcome and that she received the kind of support she required.

For the student midwife, the opportunity to carry out the total care of a patient was a valuable learning experience, producing a greater understanding of the various requirements of both mother and baby. The student obtained a great sense of satisfaction from being able to identify problems, plan the appropriate intervention and achieve a successful outcome.

Disadvantages of the model for nursing

One of the main disadvantages associated with the application of the model for nursing was the very limited time at our disposal to absorb the facts associated with the model and to rethink an approach to the patient in terms of ALs. The attempt to convey to the student the information on the model for nursing and the particular approach was not accomplished to our complete satisfaction. It soon became clear that nursing plans for actual and potential problems and daily care of mother and baby would be required. To draw up such plans would require a lot of time, trial runs and alterations in the light of feedback. A deterrent to implementing the model for nursing or any other style involving the nursing process is the additional time required to collect and record the appropriate data.

The recent introduction of a $37\frac{1}{2}$ hour working week has created difficulties regarding continuity of patient care. During the project, the student midwife had two days off and it was not possible for another student to have sufficient in-depth knowledge of the model for nursing to maintain the same level of contact with the patient. Education of the total nursing staff would be necessary to achieve the full application of the model for nursing.

When the assessment form was used for two patients prior to the actual project, it was difficult to ask personal questions in a four-bedded unit with only screens for privacy. It would therefore be advantageous to have privacy when carrying out the initial assessment.

The assessment form would require some additional headings for use in midwifery. The husband's occupation, for example, may have significance in relation to the care of the patient. If it is in the lower range, or his continuity of employment is uncertain, this may affect the relationship between husband and wife, thereby putting the baby into the 'at risk' category. Such knowledge enables the mother to be given advice regarding what supplementary benefits may be available, and alerts the health visitor to give adequate support in the postnatal period. Similarly, the patient should be asked if there is a history of any genetic disorder in the family. A section on prenatal care would be required, since it is important to have certain information prior to labour and the birth of the baby. Some details regarding length of labour, type of delivery and condition of baby at birth should also be recorded on the assessment form. Both prenatal and postnatal data should be recorded under these headings, since the section for 'expressing sexuality' does not seem to be appropriate for this information.

Conclusion

When we first embarked on this project we were not sure what to expect, or what benefits we would derive from the exercise. It took more time than we anticipated, but we enjoyed the challenge and learned a great deal which we hope to develop in the future. The student midwife found the exercise very rewarding and stimulating, stating that she found it a 'real learning experience'.

The patient also derived a great deal from the project and was very satisfied with the way in which her needs were met. A large factor in the implementation of the model for nursing would be the education of all the staff, which not only would take time but commitment on the part of everyone.

The application of the model for nursing to one patient was an interesting exercise but cannot in any way be regarded as an extended trial. This would necessitate using a number of patients over a considerable period of time, with regular reviews. However, given the right conditions, we would like to see such a trial carried out.

Figures to this chapter start on page 72.

Patient Assessment Form

Date of admission 3/9

Date of assessment 3/9

Surname Temple

Forenames Catherine

Male [ ]

Female [✓]

Age 22

Date of birth

Single/Married/Widowed [✓ over Married]

Other

Prefers to be addressed as

Mrs. Temple

Address of usual residence 267 Harris Road

Type of accommodation 2 roomed flat with outside toilet, no bathroom.

Family/Others at this residence Husband

Next of kin Name Charles Temple

Address as above.

Relationship Husband

Tel. no. none

Significant others Relatives/Dependents Parents of husband and wife alive : good relationship with in-laws.

Helpers Mother and sister willing to help after Mrs. Temple returns home from hospital.

Visitors Mostly relations.

Occupation Shop assistant.

Religious beliefs and relevant practices Roman Catholic.

Patient's perception of current health status Feels very well.

Reason for admission/referral Awaiting delivery of her baby

Medical diagnosis Pregnancy : term + 4 days. For induction of labour.

Past medical history Laparotomy for ectopic pregnancy.

Allergies none.

Significant life crises Married 2 years ago. Birth of baby.

Fig. 6.1 Patient Assessment Form: biographical, health and AL data (mother)

Assessment of Activities of Living

Date 3/9

Patient's problems
(actual/potential)
(p)= potential

AL	Usual routines: what he/she can and cannot do independently	
● Maintaining a safe environment	Has to be tidy with only 2 rooms; fitted kitchen and good hot water supply from central heating. Knowledgeable about safety in the house and the importance of hand washing.	
● Communicating	Adequate vocabulary: distinct speech: quiet, not very forthcoming: pleasant. 5/9 more responsive: at ease with staff. 6/9 Initiated discussion about baby care.	● (P) lack of bonding.
● Breathing	Doesn't smoke and has no breathing problems.	
● Eating and drinking	Height: 1.6m Weight: 64 kg Attends dentist regularly. No false teeth. Has a good appetite and eats a well balanced diet. Takes alcohol occasionally, but abstained during pregnancy.	
● Eliminating	Micturition normal. Bowels opened each day.	
● Personal cleansing and dressing	Very particular about personal hygiene. Looks fresh and attractive. Visits mother for bath twice weekly.	● (P) Infection
● Controlling body temperature	Normal.	
● Mobilising	Typical maternity gait 3/9 Was able to get up to toilet 8 hrs. after birth of baby and continued to walk round ward area at will, except during rest periods.	
● Working and playing	Shop assistant until 2 months ago: intends to return to work after maximum maternity leave as husband unable to find employment. Enjoys walking and reading	
● Expressing sexuality	Very relaxed in husband's company. Pregnancy unplanned. 8/9 confident and loving when handling baby.	● lack of knowledge about family planning.
● Sleeping	Normally a good sleeper: lately disturbed 9/9 Now sleeping well apart from feeding baby during night.	
● Dying		

Assessment of Activities of Living

Date 3/9

Patient's problems
(actual/potential)
(p)= potential

AL	Usual routines: what he/she can and cannot do independently Baby Laura Temple.	
● Maintaining a safe environment	Can't do anything independently – totally dependent on mother. Needs a warm environment.	
● Communicating	Can cry and move body to indicate discomfort. Stops crying and looks contented after attention.	
● Breathing	Can breathe normally; no signs of distress.	● (P) Respiratory difficulties
● Eating and drinking	Baby has a good sucking reflex and is eager to feed. No regurgitation after first feed. Takes the total amount required in a 24 hr. period.	● (P) Jaundice
● Eliminating	Has passed urine and meconium.	
● Personal cleansing and dressing	Totally dependent on mother and nursing staff for general hygiene.	● (P) Infection
● Controlling body temperature	3/9 First recording of temperature normal. 9/9 Recordings within normal range.	
● Mobilising	Can move all parts of the body.	
● Working and playing		
● Expressing sexuality	Once mother had established bonding with her baby, baby snuggled into mother and appeared contented.	
● Sleeping	Slept well between feeds; no long periods of wakefulness.	
● Dying		

Fig. 6.2 Patient Assessment Form: assessment of ALs (baby)

Name: Mrs. Katherine Temple _____ Unit no.::

Date	Problem identified	a = actual / p = potential	Goal	Date commenced	Nursing action	Date discontinued	Outcome
4/9	Mother feels awkward when feeding & changing her baby.	(a)	To enable mother to feel confident when handling her baby.	4/9	Advise & demonstrate on handling & feeding baby. Stay with mother while she handles & feeds baby. Give encouragement & reassurance at every opportunity.	10/9	Mother now confident & relaxed when looking after baby.
5/9	Mother complained of slight intermittent abdominal pain.	(a)	To find cause and relieve symptoms.	5/9	Observations carried out 4HR. Urinary output. Lochial discharge.	6/9	Abdominal pain disappeared without any treatment.
	Infection.	(p)	To prevent infection.		Advice given re vulval toilet hand washing general hygiene. Observations on involution of uterus, lochial discharge & 4HR		No sign of any infection.
6/9	Constipation & sub involution of uterus.	(a)	To achieve involution of uterus and relieve constipation.	6/9	2 suppositories given. Advice given regarding roughage in diet.		Bowels opened, good result. Fundal height decreased by 2.5 cm.
8/9	Passed a small blood clot, per vagina.	(a)	To determine that the lochial discharge returns to normal.		Blood clot examined for membranes or placenta – negative findings. Reassurance.		No further blood clots.

Fig. 6.3 Individual postnatal care plan for mother

Name: _Mrs Catherine Temple_   Unit no.: _____

Date	Problem identified	a = actual p = potential	Goal	Date commenced	Nursing action	Date discontinued	Outcome
11/9	Anxiety about family planning.	(a)	Provide patient with information on family planning & contraception.	11/9	Discuss different methods of family planning, give leaflets and address of nearest family planning clinic.	13/9	Knowledge of family planning relieved anxiety about the future. Has decided to attend FP clinic for further advice.
11/9	Anxiety about bathing baby & making up feeds now that discharge is imminent	(a)	To produce confidence in mother when bathing baby & making up feeds.	11/9	Actual baby bath demonstration. Mother supervised bathing her own baby. Demonstration of sterilisation of equipment & making up artificial feed. Reassured that community midwife will visit her at home for first few days.		Patient feels more confident about overall care of baby.
						13/9	Patient discharged

Fig. 6.3 Individual postnatal care plan for mother (contd)

Name: Baby Laura Temple   Unit no.: _____

Date	Problem identified	a = actual p = potential	Goal	Date commenced	Nursing action	Date discontinued	Outcome
3/9	Respiratory Problems.	(A)	To maintain a clear airway.		To aspirate mucus when necessary.		Breathing normal.
5/9	Red buttocks.	(A)	To restore the skin to normal.	5/9	Careful cleansing of napkin area + application of Vaseline.	6/9	Redness of buttocks disappeared.
	Infection	(p)	To prevent infection		Daily observation of baby for infection bond care. General instructions to mother on standards of hygiene when feeding + handling baby.		Healthy baby with no sign of infection.

Fig. 6.4   Individual postnatal care plan for baby

STANDARD POSTNATAL CARE PLAN FOR MOTHER

	Name:	Unit:
AL	*Setting of goals*	*Means of achievement*
Maintaining a safe environment	Accepting atmosphere in which patient is able to voice problems about safety Confident patient able to use call system Satisfactory bonding of mother and baby	Establish rapport with patient Demonstrate call system Give support and assistance with baby care
Communicating	Patient's psychological and social needs met to her satisfaction	Relieve any anxiety about home situation by informing appropriate bodies for assistance Provide opportunity for family to visit Recognise early signs of depression
Breathing	Absence of pulmonary embolism	Deep breathing exercises
Eating and drinking	Eating appropriate diet	Ensure diet contains the necessary minerals and vitamins
Eliminating	Normal bladder function Absence of constipation	Check micturition and urinary output Give laxative when required Assist patient on first visit to toilet after birth of baby and observe that instructions on hygiene are carried out
Personal cleansing and dressing	Painless, uninfected perineum	Teach perineal hygiene Use of bidet to soothe perineum
Controlling body temperature	Absence of pyrexia	Take temperature twice daily
Mobilising	Foot exercises while in bed and early ambulation	Help patient to get out of bed; give appropriate support
Expressing sexuality (Reproductive system)	Painless, uninfected breasts Return of uterus to previous size and position.	Daily observation of breasts, lochia and fundal height
Sleeping	Rested, untired mother adapting to night wakening to attend baby	Stress importance of daytime rest periods

Fig 6.5   Standard postnatal care plan for mother

7
A study of an elderly patient in hospital
using the model for nursing

Irene Reid and Anne Blackie

Previous experience of the nursing process

Two and a half years ago the nursing officer told us about the nursing process. We attended lectures, read some literature and talked a great deal about it before deciding to try out this new method of carrying out nursing.

A central committee was formed consisting of members from each hospital in the group, and a local committee in each hospital consisting of two members from each ward.

As the main function of using the nursing process is to ensure individual planned care for each patient, the central committee developed a patient profile (Fig. 7.1, pp. 82-83) and a care plan (Fig. 7.2, p. 84) to achieve this. At that time the nursing Kardex was filed with the patients' other case-notes on discharge from hospital and was considered a legal document. We therefore had to continue writing it up as well as the two new documents. In an attempt to minimise writing we filled in the care plan in pencil and rubbed out the previous treatment and nursing instructions as these changed, before entering the current treatment and nursing instructions.

After 18 months the nursing Kardex form was discarded and the patient profile and care plan were to be filed on discharge for legal purposes. Therefore the care plan was written in ink and it is a record of all the planned care carried out during the patient's stay in hospital.

During this time the nursing staff became increasingly involved in interviewing patients to fill in the profile and from the information gained, planning individual nursing for each patient. The learners and the nursing auxiliaries were very impressed and felt that they were taking an active part in the planning of the patients' care. The doctors, physiotherapists, occupational therapists, dietitians and medical social workers all showed scepticism in the early stages but they became interested and now refer to the profile and the care plan for information.

It was on the basis of this prolonged interest that we agreed, not without hestitation and apprehension to participate in the project, and to try out the Roper, Logan and Tierney model for nursing in a geriatric ward.

Clinical setting for the patient study

The small hospital in which the study was carried out has two storeys and is in the middle of a busy city. It stands in its own grounds surrounded by very pleasant gardens.

THE UNIT

A 32 bed female geriatric assessment and rehabilitation unit was the setting for the study. It has one main area divided into two bays, one having four beds and the other five. Patients are usually admitted into this area for assessment. There are also two two-bed wards, three four-bed wards and one six-bed ward. One single room is kept in reserve for very ill or terminally ill patients. There is a locker and a wardrobe within easy access of each bed.

The unit has one large sitting room which is also used for dining purposes. It is easily reached; the corridors are wide to accommodate wheelchairs and patients walking with Zimmers. It has a colour television, and the provision of small tables permits patients to pursue their leisure activities. There are adequate toilet facilities easily accessible from the sitting room and the bed areas.

PATTERN OF THE PATIENTS' DAY

The patients' day begins around seven o'clock, breakfast being served around eight. The whole morning is taken up with washing and dressing, having treatment, and attending physio or occupational therapy as required. This period is broken with a mid-morning drink.

Lunch is served around 12.15 p.m. after which patients get ready for visitors. For those who do not have visitors, the nurses provide diversional therapy if they wish to participate.

The evening meal is served around six o'clock, after which patients decide what they are going to do for the rest of the evening and when they are going to bed.

Preparation for the study

In preparation for carrying out the patient study using the model we read *The Elements of Nursing*. It took time to think of maintaining a safe environment as carrying out activities to prevent pollution (including noise pollution), fire, accidents and infection, yet they were all very relevant to a geriatric unit.

We had previously thought of controlling body temperature as a purely physiological function and not as an activity of living. And yet everyone carries out activities to assist that function; the fact that in hospital shoulder capes and knee rugs are provided for the patients is witness to this.

Could the activity of expressing sexuality be applicable to geriatric patients? When we turned it round and began to think about the ways in which masculinity and femininity are expressed it made more sense. For example hairstyles: 'short back and sides' in the male wards, longer hair in the female wards; night attire: pyjamas in the male wards, nightdresses in the female wards; toilet bags: bold in colour and texture in the male wards, pastel shades and soft textures in the female wards. We also began to notice differences in the type of greeting given by male/female patients to their spouses and other male and female visitors and we decided that expressing sexuality was indeed applicable in a geriatric ward.

But we had even more difficulty in coming to terms with the activity of dying, yet it is the final act of living! As it transpired, the selected patient did not mention death or dying so there is no documentation for this AL. Had the subject been mentioned we would have discussed it; we now have a policy that the patient is not cut off but encouraged to express her thoughts.

Patient study

In common with most geriatric units the average age of the patients is increasing but in our remit we were asked to select a female patient in her sixties who was likely to stay for about six weeks.

SELECTION OF THE PATIENT

Mrs Reid, a short woman of medium build, was very disabled with disseminated sclerosis; she had fallen several times at home when walking, even with the help of a Zimmer aid. Her anxiety about wetting the bed at nights meant that she frequently asked her husband to take her to the toilet, sometimes twice in one hour, so that he too was exhausted. She was therefore admitted for urinary investigations, continence training and rehabilitation of her mobilising activities. We considered that she would be an ideal participant in the project.

CONSENT OF THE PATIENT

We explained the circumstances to Mr and Mrs Reid and they seemed interested. It was made clear to them that the data collected would be used in a chapter of a book. They both readily agreed and being intelligent people they enjoyed the thought of participating in this venture.

PATIENT ASSESSMENT FORM

We were pleased about the amount of useful information collected by interviewing Mrs Reid using the Patient Assessment Form (Fig. 7.3, pp. 86–87). It was especially helpful to be reminded at a glance of Mrs Reid's actual and potential problems. However, we felt that we would have liked a space for a brief description of the patient, such as 'short woman of medium build, has long brown hair in bun'; it would alert a new nurse as to what to expect on her first approach to the patient.

NURSING PLAN

We had been used to the care plan illustrated in Figure 7.2 (p. 84) and although we were not entirely satisfied with it we had difficulty in designing a plan using the activities of living as a framework. Our first attempt involved a lot of repetitious writing of the ALs as headings. This meant that information about a particular AL became separated and it was not easy to ascertain the patient's progress in carrying out a particular AL. It seemed that the only way to have sequential information was to have a separate sheet for each AL and the result is set out in Figure 7.4 (pp. 88–96).

Mrs Reid's biggest problem was urinary incontinence, and the 'eliminating' page of Figure 7.4 (p. 93) shows how and when daytime continence was achieved and the various interventions which were tried before an overnight 'dry bed' was achieved. This involved trying to ge Mrs Reid to go against all normal habit and use incontinence pads instead of asking her husband to help her to get up so often during the night. The reason for all this planning was simply that if Mr Reid did not get his sleep during the night he would not be able to care for Mrs Reid at home after discharge from hospital.

The model for nursing

We found that use of the Patient Assessment Form provided an opportunity to collect a very realistic account of Mrs Reid's previous life-style, not just about the few weeks prior to admission. Alerted to think about what patients can do for themselves, at the first interview we discovered how many personal hygiene activities she could manage to do in spite of her disabilities.

The activity of communicating is very important in a geriatric ward because many patients have facial paresis, dysphasia and aphasia, so that knowledge of their speech habits prior to such affliction is important. Similarly, knowledge of elderly people's previous orientation to time and place is important; even those who were not confused before admission, can become confused and disorientated after admission due to change of environment.

The information about Mrs Reid's previous work and play habits was very useful when talking with her; she said that she felt that all members of the nursing staff were interested in her as a person, not just as a patient.

Conclusions

We consider that trying out the model for nursing was a useful experience. The framework of the twelve ALs was particularly relevant to an elderly patient. We would like to see it used for more patients and over a longer period to find out whether the documentation is manageable, if for instance the model is tried out for all patients in a ward.

Figures to this chapter start on page 82.

Patient Profile

Name ....

SOCIAL HISTORY

Lives alone ....Yes No

If no, who with?...

Responsible relative/friend.................................

....

Pension Book Holder.......................................

Any Home problems ....

....

....

Who will do laundry? ....

COMMUNITY SERVICES

Community Nurse ....Yes No

How often? ....

Help required ....

....

Home Help ....Yes No

Details ....

Meals on Wheels ....

Social Worker ....

Other ....

....

PAST MEDICAL HISTORY/OPERATIONS ....

....

....

....

....

**WHAT DOES PATIENT SAY IS
REASON FOR ADMISSION** ....

....

....

....

....

....

PRESENT MEDICAL PROBLEMS ....

....

....

....

....

....

....

ALLERGIES...

....

MEDICATION ON ADMISSION.......................

....

....

....

....

....

DIET ....

Food or drink dislikes.....................................

....

Appetite ....

....

Swallowing ....

....

SLEEP...

How many hours?..

How many pillows?..

Sedation...

....

ELIMINATION

Bowels

How often do bowels move?............................

....

Any problems?..

....

....

Aperients..

....

....

Urinary

No problems   Frequency

Urgency   Pain

Incontinence Day/Night

Remarks...

....

....

Aids, Pads etc...

....

Fig. 7.1   Patient profile (form already in use in ward)

Record Number

HEARING
Good   Poor   Deaf
Hearing Aid   Yes No
Remarks.....................................
....
....

VISION
Good   Poor   Blind
Glasses.....................................
....
Remarks.....................................
....

ORAL
Teeth.......................................
Dentures...................................
Cleaning...................................
Out/In at night..........................
Problems..................................
....

MOBILITY
Help needed with:—
Walking   Standing   Washing
Dressing   Feeding
Out of Chair   In/Out of bed
Details.....................................
....

AID/PROSTHESES/APPLIANCE
....
....
Help required............................
....
Problems..................................
....

SMOKER   Yes No
How many?...............................

INTERESTS.............................
....
....
....
....

GENERAL APPEARANCE
Obese   Thin   Dehydrated
Acutely ill   Emaciated
Remarks.....................................
....
....

MENTAL STATE
Orientated   Confused
Anxious   Withdrawn
Disturbed
Semi-conscious   Unconscious
Observations.............................
....
....
....

SKIN
Broken areas   Rash   Clear
Oedematous   Bruising
Jaundiced
Describe....................................
....
....

SPEECH
Clear   Aphasic
Difficulty with words
Difficulty with sentences
....
....
....

ADDITIONAL OBSERVATIONS
....
....
....
....
....

Completed by............................
Grade..
Information given by
Patient   Relative
or...

Name Mrs. Anne Reid

Age 67 yrs.

Physio Daily.

O.T. Daily.

Observations
TPR T.36.8 P.82 R.22 BP 160/90
Urinalysis — Sugar 2% Acetone +
Weight 8 st. 8 lb.

Treatment by Medical Staff and/or Investigation
M.S.U. am 15/8 ✓
Cystometry — date to be arranged.

ACTIVITIES OF DAILY LIVING in hospital.

Bath Immersion bath twice weekly using Ambulift and two nurses.

Hair Hairdresser weekly.

Shave Small growth of facial hair — to be removed as required.

Teeth Clean teeth after meals and last thing at night.

Personal hygiene Can use basin at bedside or table — Manages to wash upper body by herself but requires help of two nurses to stand while she washes groins and a nurse to wash lower body.

Dressing Manages to put on upper garments but needs help with lower garments. Two nurses to help her stand to arrange clothes.

Mobility Needs two nurses to stand. Encourage to support herself on Zimmer when standing. Unable to walk.

Toileting 2 hourly toileting day and night.

Diet Discontinued Diabetic

Feeding Self

Sleep Goes to bed between 9 + 10 p.m. Poor sleeper — needs night sedative.

INDIVIDUAL PROBLEMS | NURSING ACTION

Bowel Movements

Date	1	2	3	4	5	6	7	8	9	10	11	12	13	14	15
APT															
	16	17	18	19	20	21	22	23	24	25	26	27	28	29	30	31
APT															

Fig. 7.2   Care plan (form already in use in ward)

Figure 7.3 follows on pages 86—87.

Patient Assessment Form

Date of admission 14/8   Date of assessment 14/8

Surname Reid   Forenames Anne

Male ☐   Age [67]   Single/Married✓/Widowed   Prefers to be addressed as
Female ✓   Other   Mrs. Reid

Date of birth

Address of usual residence

    14 Adamstow Road.

Type of accommodation   Semi-detached house: upstairs and downstairs.

Family/Others at this residence   Husband

Next of kin   Name   John Reid   Address as above

              Relationship   Husband   Tel. no. 336 9813

Significant others   Relatives/Dependents One sister in Australia. No dependents.

              Helpers   Five days a week private home help.

              Visitors   None.

Occupation   Retired domestic science teacher.

Religious beliefs and relevant practices   Church of Scotland.

Patient's perception of current health status   Well aware of health situation.

Reason for admission/referral   Falls due to D.S. ? Fracture of humerus.

Medical diagnosis   Disseminated sclerosis.

Past medical history   Rheumatic fever as child. D.S. diagnosed 1955.

Allergies   None   Significant life crises Diagnosis - Disseminated Scl

Fig. 7.3 Patient Assessment Form: biographical, health and AL data

Assessment of Activities of Living

Date 14/8

Patient's problems
(actual/potential)
(p)= potential

AL	Usual routines: what he/she can and cannot do independently	

● Maintaining a safe environment — Toilet and shower downstairs. Wall rail in toilet. Sits in chair to wash, dress and cook.

● (P) Risk of falling.

● Communicating — Good conversationalist, able to talk about her feelings. Knowledgeable about disseminated sclerosis. Outgoing and comfortable with eye contact. Hearing satisfactory. Wears glasses for reading. Concentration deteriorating. Depressed at times

● (P) Increased depression.

● Breathing — R 22   BP. 160/90
Non smoker but prone to respiratory infection.

● (P) Respiratory infection.

● Eating and drinking — Weight 60 kg. Height not recorded. Has own teeth. Breakfast 8am: cereal, tea and toast. Light lunch midday. Main cooked meal 6–7 pm. Enjoys cooking. Occasional alcoholic drink. Does not drink water. Hot chocolate in bed around 9–10 pm.

● Eliminating — Urine 2% sugar. Acetone +. Incontinent of urine, dribbles most of time. Uses Kanga pads and pants day and night. Bowels used to be regular every other day after breakfast but lately constipation has been troublesome.

● Dribbling incontinence.
● Constipation.

● Personal cleansing and dressing — Cleans own teeth morning and evening. All-over wash each am. Showers twice weekly helped by home help. Can wash upper part, needs help for lower half. Hairdresser weekly. Wears blouses and trousers. Difficulty in fastening buttons and zips. Needs help to remove facial hair. Skin intact.

● Dependent for washing back, dressing.
● (P) Pressure sores.

● Controlling body temperature — T 36·8   P 82
Does not like too much heat.

● Mobilising — Up to a week prior to admission walked with zimmer. Managed stairs until recently – came downstairs on buttocks. Uses rope ladder to pull herself into sitting position in bed.

● Increasing immobility.

● Working and playing — Was domestic science teacher. Retired at 42, ill health. Played hockey in youth. Enjoys cooking, reading, writing letters, watching TV.

● Expressing sexuality — Comfortable with femininity. Positive warm relationship with husband.

● Sleeping — Goes to bed 9–10 pm, usually asleep in ½ hour. Wakes frequently. Worried about incontinence. Sometimes gets husband up twice in one hour. Rises around 7 am. Now on sleeping pills.

● Frequent wakening.

● Dying

Nursing Plan *maintaining a Safe Environment.*

Problem(s)	Goal	Nursing Intervention	Evaluation
14/8 Risk of falling	No falling	14/8 Keep environment trip free. Encourage activities which strengthen leg muscles.	24/8 No trauma. 4/9 No trauma. 16/9 No trauma.

Fig. 7.4 Nursing plan

Nursing Plan *communicating*.

Problem(s)	Goal	Nursing Intervention	Evaluation
14/8 (p) Depression	no continuous depression.	15/8 See that Mrs. Reid is where she wants to be – IN, bedside. See that books and writing paper are nearby. When in sitting room encourage her to join in conversation.	14/8 Seems a bit anxious. 21/8 Very pleased with progress in mobilising. 23/8 Very distressed about incontinence at night. 27/8 Happier and relaxed because she had slept better. 29/8 morale high. 2/9 Pleased about going home but apprehensive. 9/9 Very bright.

Nursing Plan Breathing.

Problem(s)	Goal	Nursing Intervention	Evaluation
14/8 (p) Respiratory infection.	No respiratory infection.	14/8 Teach patient deep breathing and foot exercises X 3 after meals. 11/9 Encourage patient to continue exercises.	11/9 Free from respiratory infection.

Fig. 7.4 Nursing plan (contd)

Nursing Plan Eating and Drinking.

Problem(s)	Goal	Nursing Intervention	Evaluation
	maintain current weight 60 kg.	14/8 Supervise Mrs. Reid feeding self at table with normal diet. 15/8 Discuss with Mrs. Reid overnight fasting for blood sugar. 16/8 Give breakfast after blood sugar taken. 17/8 Diabetic diet. 18/8 Give faecal softener daily. Encourage to take bran, fresh fruit and high fibre diet. Introduce to dietitian. 21/8 Give oral hypoglycaemics.	15/8 Ate all meals. 16/8 Fasted overnight.

Nursing Plan Eliminating.

Problem(s)	Goal	Nursing Intervention	Evaluation
14/8 Excreting sugar and acetone in urine.	Excreting sugar and acetone - free urine.	14/8 Test urine. 15/8 Test urine. 17/8 Test urine before meals. 24/8 Test urine 7 am. and 5 pm. 28/8 Teach patient to test urine.	14/8 Sugar 2% Acetone. 15/8 Sugar 2% Acetone. 24/8 Urine free of sugar and acetone. 28/8 Urine free of sugar and acetone.
17/8 Constipation.	Return to previous bowel habit – every other day after breakfast.	17/8 Insert two suppositories, examine result. 18/8 Insert two glycerol suppositories, examine result. Give phosphate enema. Give arachis oil enema.	17/8 No result from suppositories. No faeces in lower rectum, hard faeces higher up. 18/8 Faeces lower. No result from suppositories. No result from phosphate enema. Hard, dry faeces after arachis oil enema. 14/9 Bowels open most days.

Fig. 7.4 Nursing plan (contd)

Nursing Plan Eliminating.

Problem(s)	Goal	Nursing Intervention	Evaluation
14/8 Dribbling urinary incontinence.	Daytime continence, cope with night-time incontinence.	14/8 Fill in incontinence chart by bed. Toilet 2 hourly – even hours during day. 18/8 Maxi pads and pants day and night. Continue chart. Prepare for cystometry at 2 pm. 19/8 " 22/8 Continue but toilet on demand. 25/8 Waken about 2.30 am., toilet. " " 6.30 am., " 26/8 Continue but standard maxi plus pads at night. Note if bed is wet at 2.30 am., 6.30 am. 28/8 Continue but at night maxi pad and ½ Kanga pad. 30/8 As above but with incontinence pad under buttocks during night. 7/9 As at 30/8.	18/8 Cystometry cancelled. 19/8 Cystometry – bladder has small volume and is unstable. 22/8 Continent during day on 1½ hourly toileting. 26/8 Bed wet at 2.30. 27/8 Only pad wet at 2.30 and 6.30. 28/8 Pad and bed wet 2.30. Pad wet, bed dry 6.30. 30/8 Bed slightly damp at 2.30. 31/8 Dry incontinence pad and bed. 2/9 " 3/9 " 5/9 " 7/9 "

Nursing Plan Personal Cleansing and Dressing.

Problem(s)	Goal	Nursing Intervention	Evaluation
14/8 Dependent for washing bathing dressing	Achievement of optimal independence for washing bathing dressing	14/8 Basin at bedside, patient can wash upper half, needs help for lower half. Help with dressing: 2 nurses to support Mrs. Reid standing while clothes are arranged.	16/8 Managing to wash and dress upper half of body. 24/8 Managed to dress with help of only one nurse. Pressure areas healthy.
(P) Pressure sores	Unblemished skin over pressure areas.	Usual intervention	

Fig. 7.4 Nursing plan (contd)

Nursing Plan *mobilising.*

Problem(s)	Goal	Nursing Intervention	Evaluation
14/8 Increasing immobility.	Increased mobility.	14/8 Two nurses to give maximum support without which Mrs. Reid cannot stand. 17/8 Prepare for X-ray of L. arm. 21/8 Give praise, encourage. Once on feet, encourage use of Zimmer aid.	16/8 Trying hard to stand with less support. 17/8 No fracture 21/8 Got up from chair, stood and moved feet a little with help from doctor and nurse. 23/8 Showing improvement 31/8 Managing to stand and take a few steps. with Zimmer aid.

Nursing Plan Sleeping.

Problem(s)	Goal	Nursing Intervention	Evaluation
14/8 Frequent wakening.	Increased sleeping time, dry bed in the morning.	14/8 Help Mrs. Reid cope with night time incontinence. Help her to believe that the problem of seepage from pads into sheet will be solved. Give sedatives 1 hour before retiral. 19/8 Continue reassurance. Change sedation. 25/8 Give double strength sedative. Report sleep pattern in detail. 30/8 Encouragement to sleep instead of asking frequently for the toilet. Explain that the pads are made to absorb urine passed during the night.	14/8 Wakening frequently sometimes more than once an hour. 16/8 Still wakening frequently 17/8 ” 18/8 ” 19/8 ” 20/8 Wakened fewer times. 21/8 ” 22/8 ” 23/8 Sleep periods longer than 1½ hours. 24/8 ” 25/8 ” 26/8 Increased sleep periods. 27/8 Further increase in sleep periods. 28/8 ” 29/8 ” 30/8 Slept well before and after 2.30 am. toileting. 31/8 ” 1/9 ” 2/9 ” 11/9 ” 13/9 Wakened a few times. 14/9 Wakened fewer times. 17/9 ” 19/9 Wakened more times. 20/9 Wakened less times. 22/9 Wakened more times.

Fig. 7.4 Nursing plan (contd)

8

A study in a medical ward
using the model for nursing

Mary Birkett Colquhoun and Agnes Fraser

Introduction

CLINICAL SETTING

The medical nursing study was undertaken in a 28-bed acute general medical ward within a large inner-city hospital. Four of the ward's five consultants specialise in specific medical fields namely haematology, cardiology, diabetes mellitus and respiratory disorders. As a result the ward has

- a great diversity of disease conditions
- a tremendous variation in patients' nursing requirements
- a wide age range of patients
- a rapid rate of patient turnover.

In design the ward retains its original Florence Nightingale style layout: 22 beds positioned in two opposing rows within the main ward area. Two single cubicles and a four-bed side ward adjoin the service corridor leading into the main ward. Toilets, bathroom and dayroom are situated at the far end of the main ward. The nursing station is based just inside the main ward.

STAFFING LEVELS

The nursing staff on day duty comprise one charge nurse, five staff nurses, one auxiliary, one orderly, plus a variable quota (minimum level five) of student and pupil nurses, including nursing degree students, shortened course for graduate students, pre-registration students and students seconded from psychiatry, mental deficiency and paediatrics.

Introducing the nursing process

THE PROBLEMS

With the aid of books and articles sister had introduced the concept of the nursing process to the ward's permanent nursing staff about a year before our involvement in this project. Much interest and enthusiasm was shown, but four problem areas became rapidly apparent when considering the feasibility of applying the nursing process in a clinical setting of the type described.

Firstly, existing hospital nursing records consisted of only the Kardex. To effect adequate documentation and implementation of the nursing process totally revised forms would have to be introduced, detailing patient assessment, identified problems and goals, proposed nursing action and consequent evaluation. Where were such forms to be obtained?

Secondly, it emerged that student and pupil nurses were not being taught in the college how to document the nursing process because there was no acknowledged standard hospital system of documentation. The onus would thus fall on ward staff to teach individual nurses how to document the nursing process.

Thirdly, given that patient allocation is an integral part of the practical application of the nursing process (in contradistinction to the system of task allocation) how could we consistently cope with the weekly fluctuations in staffing levels and the high service dependency on junior nurses who are still learning? Furthermore how could we realistically subdivide a Nightingale style ward such that each nurse worked primarily in a given area, but was not deterred from assisting elsewhere when necessary?

Fourthly, nursing staff were keen to leave patients' nursing records at each bed-side for ease of access by staff and to facilitate recording/planning by each individual nurse. Where and how were we to keep the nursing records and how could we avoid problems relating to ease of access?

THE SOLUTIONS

Nursing records for use in implementing the nursing process were devised by ward staff, taking into account the information sought by nursing staff and the reviewed successes and failings of systems practised elsewhere. Duplication of these specially designed forms was undertaken by the hospital to suit our needs.

A ward folder was compiled detailing the principles of the

nursing process and providing examples of its application in a medical ward setting. Time was set aside to formally teach all nursing staff who would be working in the ward at the time of 'changeover'. All were given ample opportunity to question the method and air grievances. Following on from a pre-determined date all new patients were admitted to the ward by sister or staff nurse employing nursing process methods. Bed positions were organized such that all patients admitted under the 'new' system were nursed in adjacent beds and initially cared for by sister or one of the staff nurses. Other members of staff were thus able to study and observe implementation of the nursing process. As more and more patients were admitted, so relatively junior nurses were personally introduced to the method of patient care and given responsibility for employing the nursing process. Within approximately three weeks the nursing process was fully operational in the ward.

At the start of each day shift nurses were allocated specific patients for the remainder of the shift. Fluctuations in staffing levels admittedly varied the responsibility accorded each nurse, but level of training and extent of experience was always borne in mind and whenever possible, day-to-day consistency of patient allocation was practised. No major difficulties have emerged to date. In point of fact it was surprising how quickly nurses adapted to using the nursing process and responded positively to its inherent responsibilities.

Clinically subdividing a Nightingale style ward posed no major problems either. In general, nurses care for patients in adjacent beds. Practical assistance (for example, with lifting and turning patients) is sought by the individual nurse as and when required. Supervision and guidance by sister or staff nurse was always ongoing.

Eventually ward staff resorted to purchasing plastic folders best suited to their needs. The hospital provided bulldog clips and nursing records were subsequently clipped to the ends of the beds.

Patients are aware that these folders contain information relating to themselves as individuals: some make use of them reading the details and making pertinent comments! Access to this information by other health service personnel is sought via sister or staff nurse. There has not been a problem of patients reading other patients' records and the only visitors observed to read patients' nursing records are those encouraged to do so by the individual patients themselves. If it were deemed necessary to withhold information from a patient about his diagnosis or some aspect of his treatment (at the discretion of relatives/medical staff/nursing staff), then relevant information is carefully omitted from the nursing records.

The patient study

INTRODUCTION

Having spent a year contemplating the nursing process and trying to envisage its application in a medical ward setting, all thoughts were nursing process orientated when the editors sought our participation in this project.

The brief was to select a male patient between the ages of 20–50 years with a medical haematological disorder and, by using the model for nursing described in *The Elements of Nursing*, compile a patient study.

After much thought and deliberation we chose John, a 48-year-old works manager, known to have myeloma and admitted to the ward on 8th September following routine attendance at the haematology outpatient clinic. Permission to compile this study was given by the patient's relatives.

John had been diagnosed as having myeloma in June of that year following a two-month history of tiredness, anorexia and weight loss. During the pre-diagnosis period John was referred by his general practitioner to hospital for investigation, but pressure of work and pre-arranged business trips had led him to decline admission. It was following his return from a trip overseas, that John became sufficiently distressed by his worsening lethargy and weight loss to accept referral to hospital.

Trephine biopsy confirmed the suspected diagnosis and John was referred to this hospital's haematologists for future care. Over the following two months John had several admissions to hospital to receive cytotoxic chemotherapy and, on one occasion, to undergo renal dialysis.

The ensuing documentation details John's progress over a period dating from the time of his admission to the ward until his relatively sudden, but not altogether unexpected, death, 25 days later.

On admission John clearly looked ill and very unhappy. In the six months since he had moved north from England to his present job he had had to contend with several hospital admissions, the knowledge that he had a malignant disease and the ever increasing restrictions imposed by a worsening health status. Arrangements enabling his wife and family to join him in their new home had only recently been completed. Now to complicate matters further he had developed a left basal pneumonia.

The first assessment was undertaken on that day of admission (Figs 8.1 and 8.2, pp. 100-101). Over the following few weeks John's condition altered markedly although the day-to-day variation in health status appeared slight. This posed difficulties in terms of knowing how frequently to reassess the activities of living. For the purposes of documentation, storage and easy reading we believed that all of the twelve activities of living required to be reassessed, and not just individual ALs, as change was noted. To that end, therefore, we undertook a total of four assessments, each denoting a clearly identifiable change in John's condition (Figs 8.2, 8.4, 8.6 and 8.8).

DOCUMENTATION

The four assessments mentioned above are contained in the following set of documents which form the substance of the patient study. Each assessment is followed by a statement of problems, goals and plans (Figs 8.3, 8.5, 8.7 and 8.9).

Patient Assessment Form

Date of admission 8 Sept.   Date of assessment 8 Sept.

Surname Black   Forenames John

Male [✓]   Age   Single/*Married*/Widowed   Prefers to be addressed as
Female [ ]   [48]   Other   John
                   Date of birth

Address of usual residence   2, Elmwood Terrace.

Type of accommodation   Ground Floor. Terraced house.

Family/Others at this residence Wife   Son   Daughter

Next of kin   Name   Mary Black.   Address   Same address.

                 Relationship Wife.   Tel. no.   —

Significant others   Relatives/Dependents   All other relatives live in Sheffield.

                     Helpers

                     Visitors

Occupation   Civil Engineer   Works Manager

Religious beliefs and relevant practices   Protestant

Patient's perception of current health status   Knows that he has cancer.

Reason for admission/referral   Found to have (L) basal pneumonia on routine attendance at
                                Out-patient clinic.

Medical diagnosis   Myeloma   Left basal pneumonia.

Past medical history   Myeloma (diagnosed 3 months prior to admission).

Allergies   None known. | Significant life crises Family moved to present
                                          | address from Sheffield only 1 month ago.

Fig. 8.1 Patient Assessment Form: biographical and health data

Assessment of Activities of Living ①

Date 8 Sept.

AL	Usual routines: what he/she can and cannot do independently	Patient's problems (actual/potential) (p)= potential
● Maintaining a safe environment	Normally independent. Currently grudgingly aware of severe health limitations on ALs. Listless, lethargic, weak, drowsy.	● (P) Risk of self-injury.
● Communicating	Normally pleasant mannered, articulate, intelligent. Pronounced Sheffield accent. Short, curt responses to questions. Anxious; unhappy; slow to respond. Wife conveying required information.	● Diminished verbal response. ● Anxiety / Depression ● Accent
● Breathing	Smoked 20/30 cigarettes / day. Recently reduced to 3/day. Dyspnoea; troublesome cough; pain on coughing; expectorating tenacious purulent secretions.	● Cough ● Infected sputum ● Pain ● Dyspnoea ● Cigarette smoking
● Eating and drinking	Appetite good until illness diagnosed; poor since. Little to eat or drink past few days. Thin; recent weight loss; mildly dehydrated; tongue dry and furred. Dentition: lower – extremely poor state / caries; upper – absent.	● Anorexia ● Dehydration ● Poor dentition ● (P) Oral infection
● Eliminating	No urinary or bowel problems prior to illness. Bowels moved once/day. 3 months ago – renal failure treated by renal dialysis. Now urinary frequency – approx 1 glassful / hour Intermittent constipation.	● (P) Renal failure ● (P) Renal infection ● (P) Constipation
● Personal cleansing and dressing	Normally independent, well groomed. Perspiring profusely. Settled into bed wearing outdoor clothing. Unable/unwilling to care for personal hygiene and dressing. Wife assisted with putting on of pyjamas.	● Inability / unwillingness to care for self. ● Excessive perspiration
● Controlling body temperature	Temp re. 35·8° C Skin warm to touch. Excessive perspiration.	● (P) Dehydration
● Mobilising	Fit and active until illness diagnosed; lacking in energy since. Past 2 weeks particularly listless and lethargic. Brought to ward in wheelchair. Unable to walk more than a few yards because of fatigue and dyspnoea.	● Immobility ● (P) Pressure sores ● DVT ● Exacerbation of chest infection
● Working and playing	Worked up until admission, latterly in a very limited capacity approx. 1 hour/day. Worked abroad for many years. April moved from Sheffield to new job in Scotland. Wife and family flitted into new house Aug. No relatives nearby.	
● Expressing sexuality		
● Sleeping	Sleeps well 9/10 hours/night. Recently extremely tired. Sleeping a lot during the day.	
● Dying	Patient, wife, parents all know he has cancer. Up until now unwilling to allow ill-health to interfere with plans or life style.	● (P) Non acceptance of diagnosis

Fig. 8.2   First assessment of ALs

Maintaining a Safe Environment   8 September

Problem   •(P) Risk of self-injury
Goal   Prevent self-injury
Plan   Position   bed/chair close to nursing station
              cot sides on bed
              table front attached to chair

Communicating

Problems   •Diminished verbal response • Anxiety, depression
              •Accent
Goals   Anticipate and identify needs
              Seek solutions to problems
              Aim to minimise anxiety
Plan   Close observation
              Consistent nurse allocation to promote continuity of care
              Speak clearly, avoid technical terminology
              Provide information/explanations in advance of all procedures
              Maximise use of non-verbal communication
              Chat to wife to identify fears and problems
              Involve other hospital personnel in seeking solutions to problems

Breathing

Problems   •Cough • Infected sputum •Pain • Dyspnoea
              • Cigarette smoking
Goals   Infection-free respiratory tract
              Alleviate pain and discomfort
              Reduce number of cigarettes smoked
Plan   2 hourly position change to prevent accumulation of secretions
              Head and chest well supported, raised on several pillows
              Bed table across bed to lean on
              Support chest during coughing spasms
              Teach and encourage deep breathing and expectoration
              Sputum carton within reach
              Discourage smoking
              Minimise patient effort in all ALs
              Daily sputum specimen to bacteriology
              Administer antibiotics as prescribed
              Chest physiotherapy

Fig. 8.3 Problems, goals, plans (following first assessment of ALs)

Eating and Drinking

Problems
- Anorexia • Dehydration • Poor dentition
- (P) Oral infection

Goals
Return to normal appetite and eating patterns
evidenced by weight gain, normal skin turgor and
good urinary output
moist odour-free mouth, clean lower dentition

Plans
Small, nourishing, well presented meals
Food — soft, not too hot or spicy
Assist with feeding as and when necessary
Weigh twice weekly
Determine what patient enjoys drinking (water, tea)
Aim to assist patient drink ≥ 150 mls fluid/hour
Accurately record fluid input and output
Assist patient clean his teeth after meals and rinse mouth
with mouthwash solution
Swab oral mucosa twice weekly

Eliminating

Problems
- (P) Renal failure • (P) Renal infection • (P) Constipation

Goals
Prevent renal failure and infection by ensuring adequate
hydration and reporting to doctors immediate onset of
associated abnormalities. Return to normal bowel habit.

Plans
Accurately record all fluid input and output
Test all urine with multistix
Send daily M.S.U. to Bacteriology.
24 hour urine collections for creatinine clearance and calcium
Ensure diet has adequate roughage e.g. bran, vegetables
Administer aperients as prescribed
Assist patient to sit on commode or wheel to toilet
Obtain stool specimens for F.O.B. testing
Record all bowel motions on chart

Personal Cleansing and Dressing

Problems
- Inability/unwillingness to care for self
- Excessive perspiration

Goals
Assist patient cater for own hygiene needs
without incurring distress, anxiety or embarrassment.
Clean, dry, intact skin.

Plans
See over/

Plans
    Daily bed bath / big bath
    Sponge down skin with soap and water as necessary
    Change pyjamas and bed linen immediately they become damp
    Assist patient shave daily
    Attend to hair and nails
    Ensure privacy and appreciation of modesty and independence
    (unable to use sheepskin in bed because of patient's excessive
    perspiration and need for frequent change of bed linen.)

Controlling Body Temperature

Problem
    ● (P) Dehydration

see AL of eating and drinking

Mobilising

Problems
    ● Immobility ● (P) pressure sores ● DVT
    ● Exacerbation of chest infection

Goals
    Prevent development of pressure sores and problems
    associated with immobility e.g. DVT

Plans
    2 hourly position change
    Correct body alignment at all times
    Passive limb movements when altering position
    Encourage active limb movements
    Elevate legs on stool when patient seated in chair
    Sit on air cushion when seated in chair or upright in bed
    Ensure sheets are dry and free from wrinkles
    Ensure skin kept clean and dry
    Ensure patient lifted correctly – using Australian lift
    when patient in bed
    Assist patient to take short walk morning and evening
    (anti-embolism stockings not worn because of excessive perspiration)

Dying

Problem
    ● (P) non-acceptance of nature of disease.

Goals
    Encourage patient to talk about his health and become
    more accepting of actual/potential short/long term
    implications

Plan
    Aim to establish good rapport with patient.
    Talk openly about problems

Fig. 8.3 Problems, goals, plans (contd)

Assessment of Activities of Living ②

AL	Usual routines: what he/she can and cannot do independently	Patient's problems (actual/potential) (p)= potential
● Maintaining a safe environment	As 8/9. Now also dizzy, confused, increasingly drowsy, disorientated in time, place and person. Totally dependent.	● (P) Risk of self-injury.
● Communicating	Slow to respond. Conscious level dropped due to DF 118 given I.m. Prognosis discussed with wife.	● Decreased conscious level. ● Wife told prognosis.
● Breathing	Dyspnoea. Cough with purulent secretions. Pain if lying on right side.	● Pain. ● Cough. ● Infected sputum.
● Eating and drinking	Nil orally due to diminished conscious level. Dehydrated. Tongue dry and furred. Poor lower dentition. Absent upper dentition.	● Dehydration. ● Poor dentition. ● (P) Oral infection.
● Eliminating	Incontinent of urine and faeces.	● Incontinence. ● (P) Renal failure. ● (P) Renal infection.
● Personal cleansing and dressing	Dependent on nursing staff. Unable to care for personal hygiene	● Inability to care for self. ● Excessive perspiration.
● Controlling body temperature	Temperature 36.8° C. Excessive perspiration	● Pyrexia. ● Dehydration.
● Mobilising	Decreasing conscious level hence continuous bedrest. Skin becoming increasingly red over pressure areas.	● Immobility. ● (P) Pressure sores. ● (P) DVT ● (P) Exacerbation of chest infection.
● Working and playing	As 8/9	
● Expressing sexuality		
● Sleeping	As 8/9	
● Dying	As 8/9	

Fig. 8.4 Second assessment of ALs

Maintaining a Safe Environment   12 September

Problem   • (P) Risk of self-injury
Goals   } as 8/9
Plan

Communicating

Problems   • Decreased conscious level.
                 • Wife told prognosis. Has difficulty in visiting because of children;
                   no friends locally.
Goals   Raise conscious level.
                  Increase wife's visiting and communication with husband.
Plan   Administer Narcan as prescribed.
                 Advise wife to contact relatives in Sheffield.
                 Refer to social worker, doctors and sister
                 Offer to accommodate in hospital.
                 Allow visiting at any time.

Breathing

Problems   • Pain   • Cough   • Infected sputum.
Goals   Alleviate pain and discomfort.
                 Infection-free respiratory tract.
Plan   As for 8/9
                 plus: naso-pharyngeal suction as necessary.
                 Refer to physiotherapist.
                 Obtain sputum specimens via "trap" with suction.
                 Administer analgesia as prescribed.
                 Avoid positioning on (R) side.

Eating and Drinking

Problems   • Dehydration   • Poor dentition   • (P) Oral infection
Goals   Adequate hydration evidenced by normal skin turgor and
                 good urinary output.
                 Moist, odour-free, infection-free mouth.
                 Clean lower dentition.
Plan   Intra-venous infusion carefully monitored to give 3 litres per day
                 as prescribed.
                 Cleanse mouth and teeth 2 hourly using water and swab sticks.
                 Give Nystatin suspension if conscious level permits swallowing.

Fig. 8.5 Problems, goals, plans (following second assessment of ALs)

Eliminating

Problems   • (P) Renal failure   • (P) Renal infection   • Incontinence

Goals   Prevent renal failure and infection as 8/9.
maintain clean, dry skin.

Plan   Catheterised. Hourly urimeter recordings
and urinalysis.
24 hour urine collections.
Obtain stool specimen for culture.
Obtain stool specimen for faecal occult blood
(all bowel movements).
Wash and dry thoroughly after each episode of
faecal incontinence.
Accurately record all fluid input/output.

Personal Cleansing and Dressing

Problems   • Inability to care for self   • Excessive perspiration

Goals   maintain clean, dry, intact skin.

Plan   As 8/9

Controlling Body Temperature

Problems   • Pyrexia   • Dehydration

Goals   Prevent further increase in temperature.
maintain adequate hydration.

Plan   Tepid sponge as necessary.
Dress in loose cotton gown.

Mobilising

Problems   • Immobility   • (P) Pressure sores   • (P) DVT
• (P) Exacerbation of chest infection.

Goals   } As for 8/9 but decreased concious level
Plan   } so bedrest at all times.

Dying   As 8/9

Assessment of Activities of Living ③

Date 19 Sept.

Patient's problem
(actual/potential)
(p)= potential

AL	Usual routines: what he/she can and cannot do independently	
● Maintaining a safe environment	Attempting to climb out of bed. Weak, dizzy, confused. Disorientated	● (P) Risk of self-inju ● (P) Risk of dislodgin ● (P) Attempting to smok
● Communicating	More responsive. Less drowsy. Orientated to some extent. Slow and inappropriate responses.	● Accent. ● Explanation of care and proced
● Breathing	As 12/9 but more conscious so suctioning not required.	● Pain. ● Cough. ● Infected sputum
● Eating and drinking	Now more conscious. Anorexia. IVI in situ. Poor dentition. Dry mouth and tongue.	● Anorexia. ● Dehydration. ● Poor dentition. ● (P) Oral infection
● Eliminating	Urinary catheter on free drainage. Haematuria. No further faecal incontinence.	● (P) Urinary trac infection. ● Haematuria.
● Personal cleansing and dressing	As 8/9 and 12/9. More conscious but remains dependent	● Inability to care for self.
● Controlling body temperature	Temperature 36·4° b.	
● Mobilising	Attempting to climb out of bed but too weak to stand	● (P) Risk of self-inj ● (P) Pressure sores. ● (P) DVT ● (P) Exacerbation of chest infection.
● Working and playing	As 8/9	
● Expressing sexuality		
● Sleeping	As 8/9	
● Dying	As 8/9	

Fig. 8.6   Third assessment of ALs

Maintaining a Safe Environment   19 September

Problems   • (P) Risk of self-injury.
                • (P) Risk of dislodging IVI
                • (P) Risk of causing fire due to attempting to smoke in bed.
Goals   Prevent injury.
                Maintain IVI.
                Stop smoking.
Plan   Position bed close to nursing station.
                Cot sides on bed.
                Nurse in attendance nearby.
                Remove cigarettes and matches and explain dangers.

Communicating

Problems   • Accent   • Explanation of care and procedures
Goals   As 8/9
                Achieve appreciation of circumstances
Plan   As 8/9

Breathing

                See 12/9 but no suctioning
                + 8/9

Eating and Drinking

Problems   • Anorexia   • Dehydration   • Poor dentition   • (P) Oral infection
Goals   Increase oral fluid intake so that IVI may be discontinued.
                Achieve normal eating patterns and adequate nutrition.
                Moist, clean mouth.
Plan   Encourage to drink at least one glass juice/water per hour.
                Present with small portions of soft, low sodium, 40g protein diet.
                Assist to feed self if IVI impedes use of knife and fork.
                Encourage to use mouthwash 2-hourly.

Eliminating

Problems   • Haematuria   • (P) Urinary tract infection
Goals   Infection-free urinary tract.
Plan   Daily catheter specimens of urine for culture.
                Daily urinalysis for blood.

Fig. 8.7 Problems, goals, plans (following third assessment of ALs)

Personal Cleansing and Dressing

Although more conscious remains dependent
See 8/9 and 12/9

Mobilising

Problems
- (P) Risk of self - injury
- (P) Pressure sores
- (P) DVJ
- (P) Exacerbation of chest infection

Goals
Plan
} See AL of maintaining a safe environment
} and 8/9, 12/9

Fig. 8.7   Problems, goals, plans (contd)

Assessment of Activities of Living ④

Date 30 Sept.

AL	Usual routines: what he/she can and cannot do independently	Patient's problems (actual/potential) (p)= potential
● Maintaining a safe environment	Extremely weak and drowsy. Conscious level deteriorating. Sleeping throughout most of day.	● (P) Risk of self-injury.
● Communicating	Minimal response when spoken to. No spontaneous conversation. Speech solely comprises "no" when disturbed by nursing staff e.g. when position requiring to be altered or drinks offered	● Diminished verbal response.
● Breathing	Marked deterioration; respirations laboured; using accessory muscles of respiration; showing features of air hunger. Turning head to left in jerky rhythmic movements with inspiration.	● Dyspnoea. ● Inability to expectorate.
● Eating and drinking	Totally unwilling to eat or drink; strongly protests "no" if attempts made. INT recommended; oral hygiene greatly disliked and poorly tolerated. Mouth moist. Lower dentition plaqued and difficult to clean.	● Malnourishment. ● Unwillingness to tolerate oral hygiene.
● Eliminating	Urinary catheter patent (no.1). Urinary tract infection diagnosed. Occasional minimal faecal staining on clothing; no proper bowel motions. Rectum empty.	● Urinary tract infection.
● Personal cleansing and dressing	Totally dependent. Still perspiring profusely. Requiring frequent spongedowns. Persistent changing of saturated clothing and linen greatly distressing patient.	● Total dependence. ● Excessive perspiration.
● Controlling body temperature	Temperature 37.5° C.	● Pyrexia.
● Mobilising	Total dependence for positioning. Unable to maintain position unless well supported. Skin red particularly over bony prominences. No breaks in skin.	● Total dependence. ● (P) DVT. ● (P) Pressure sores. ● Exacerbation of chest infection.
● Working and playing	No interest shown in anything. Desiring solely to sleep and be left alone.	
● Expressing sexuality		
● Sleeping	Content to sleep 24 hours a day. Awakening only when disturbed by nursing staff.	
● Dying	Extremely difficult to determine if aware of / acknowledging indications of deterioration in health status.	

Fig. 8.8 Fourth assessment of ALs

Maintaining a Safe Environment   30 September

Problem   • (P) Risk of self-injury.
Goal   Prevent self-injury.
Plan   Position chair close to nursing station.
               Table front attached to chair.
               Nurse/wife in attendance nearby.

Communicating

Problem   • Diminished verbal response.
Goal   Anticipate and identify needs. Carry out essential nursing care
               with minimal disturbance to patient.
Plan   As 8/9
               + no unnecessary disturbance of patient in view of distress caused.
               Together with doctors chat with wife regarding patient's
               worsening condition.
               Reaffirm and ensure wife understands that she can
               telephone or visit at any time.

Breathing

Problems   • Dyspnoea   • Inability to expectorate
Goals   Infection-free respiratory tract.
               Alleviate discomfort and try to determine nature, type and extent
               of any pain experienced.
               Aid expectoration of chest secretions.
               Administer O_2 therapy to ease dyspnoea.
Plan   Nurse in Buxton chair rather than in bed as former offers greater
               support to patient's position and he appears less distressed
               when seated in chair.
               Alter position 2-hourly by varying tilt angle of chair.
               Position patient's arms on table front well supported by pillows.
               Ensure head and neck well supported by pillows.
               Administer O_2 therapy by any means tolerated.
               (Despite explanations, nasal spectacles, m.b. mask, Ventimask
               all caused great distress and thus attempts to administer
               additional O_2 therapy had to be abandoned).
               Chest physiotherapy followed by naso/oro pharyngeal suction.
               (Unfortunately both procedures caused great distress to the patient,
               markedly compounding his breathing difficulties and requiring him to be
               restrained. In view of extreme distress caused and lack of appreciable
               result from either procedure, team decision taken to cease both
               chest physiotherapy and suctioning).

Fig. 8.9 Problems, goals, plans (following fourth assessment of ALs)

Eating and Drinking

Problems
• Malnourishment   • Unwillingness to tolerate oral hygiene.

Goals
Adequate hydration.
Moist, clean, fresh-smelling mouth.

Plan
Accept patient's refusal/inability to eat or drink, and concentrate
on hydrating him by other means.
Ensure IVI monitored closely and fluids infused
at prescribed rate.
Explain to patient the importance of maintaining
a moist, clean mouth.
Attempt to cleanse tongue, teeth and oral mucosa 2 hourly
using water and soft swab sticks.

Eliminating

Problem
• Urinary tract infection.

Goal
Infection-free urinary tract.

Plan
Chlorhexidine 1:5000 bladder washouts twice daily.
Daily catheter specimen of urine to Bacteriology.

Personal Cleansing and Dressing

Problems
• Total dependence   • Profuse perspiration

Goal
Cater for patient's hygiene needs and dressing
without incurring distress, anxiety or embarrassment.

Plan
Daily bed/chair bath.
Sponge down skin with soap and water
as necessary.
Shave daily.
Attend to hair and nails.
Dress patient in one-piece gown to minimise distress
caused by frequent change of clothing.

Controlling Body Temperature

Problem   • Pyrexia

Goal   Reduction of pyrexia

Plan   Tepid sponge patient when sponge downs required.
Dress patient in loose cotton gown.
Lightweight cotton sheet over legs
to preserve modesty.
Quiet fan positioned close to patient, but
outwith his reach.

Mobilising

Problems   • Total dependence
       • (P) Pressure sores
       • (P) DVT
       • (P) Exacerbation of chest infection

Goals
Plan   } As 8/9 except that patient now nursed continually in
Buxton chair; no attempts made at mobilisation.

Dying

Patient's condition continued to deteriorate
and he died on 2 October.

Fig. 8.9 Problems, goals, plans (contd)

Comments on the study

INITIAL REACTIONS TO THE PROJECT

When we were approached by the editors to take part in this project our first reactions were those of interest and enthusiasm. However, we also experienced some doubts as to how we would set about it, and about problems which might be encountered in its completion. Nonetheless, we agreed to apply the model for nursing to the care of one patient, and in doing so we did indeed meet a few difficulties.

One potential problem which the editors had envisaged was that of contributors adapting established approaches to nursing care in order to use the model. However, having read *The Elements of Nursing* we found the concept of ALs relatively easy to grasp. Unfortunately, our difficulties began when we attempted to apply the model in a practical setting.

Problems also arose in using the Patient Assessment Form itself, and in developing a suitable nursing care plan, a task which we found rather tricky. We also experienced some difficulty with assessment of the activities of living, as the headings on the form were new to us, and we each had differing ideas as to which pieces of information should be included under which heading. Details of these problems will be outlined later.

In short, then, we approached the project enthusiastically, but somewhat cautiously. During the completion of the task we encountered several problems and difficulties, mainly with documentation and with using ALs. However, for the most part, we enjoyed trying out this model.

DIFFICULTIES OF DOCUMENTATION

One of the first problems arising in considering the practical application of the nursing process is that of how best to document the stages of assessment, planning, implementation, and evaluation.

The Patient Assessment Form in this study provides a means of recording assessment data and identifying problems. However, we were requested to develop our own method of then documenting goals and plans for care. We decided that, in order to ensure that problems identified from assessment were solved, a care plan stating goals and outlining the nursing care required to meet these, was necessary. For this we used a separate sheet attached to each of the four forms for assessment of ALs.

Unfortunately, we found the addition of a further sheet to incorporate goals and plans led to a second problem. The paperwork involved became increasingly bulky as new forms for assessment of all ALs were added when changes took place in John's condition. Obviously, frequent reassessment and evaluation were necessary in order to update the care plan

appropriately, but the question then arose of how these changes could be most easily and concisely recorded. Updating the problem list on this document required completion of the whole thing, rather than amending or adding to an existing problem sheet. We felt this was unnecessarily repetitive and time-consuming, as well as adding to the bulkiness of the total records. As an example, during our study John's ability to maintain a safe environment varied very little, so that the original assessment data did not require to be altered much when we reassessed him. Thus much of the information was duplicated as we filled in the same points under that heading at each assessment. On the other hand, it was necessary to complete a new form in order to record a significant change in the other ALs such as 'mobilising', for example.

The difficulty of how best to record change is by no means unique to this model. However, we felt that by having a separate assessment form and then listing problems in addition to goals and plans on the nursing care plan, small changes could be recorded and new problems could be added to this plan on a daily basis. The problems of time-wasting and bulkiness might then be reduced, yet a record of the patient's current status would be maintained. Naturally, significant change in several ALs would merit the completion of a fresh assessment form, as the status of the patient might change considerably and complete reappraisal of his care be required.

Although assessment of the patient was a continuous, ongoing process, we felt that in our study significant change requiring the completion of a new form took place on four occasions, and for this reason we have included these assessments only.

COMMENTS ON THE FORM

In the previous discussion, several points arose in relation to the Patient Assessment Form itself.

We have already mentioned the difficulty of documenting goals and plans, but the recording of assessment information also presented problems. Firstly, we found the space provided for recording data under each AL was rather small. This led to the possibility of some details being missed through lack of space or the form becoming illegible! However, we also felt that this problem may also have been at least partly caused by our own inexperience in using the AL headings and in deciding which pieces of information were most relevant.

Nonetheless, our difficulties increased as we tried to list problems for each AL. Space for this was extremely limited and, whereas some ALs had few related problems, others had too many to fit easily into the corresponding space (for example, see Fig. 8.2, p. 101 — the ALs of 'breathing' and 'eating and drinking'). Hence the suggestion of a separate page for listing problems, and stating goals and plans. This would leave more space on the assessment form for information related to ALs.

Lastly, we found that the ALs proved very useful for ensuring comprehensive, thorough assessment. Because of this many pieces of information about the patient were collected, and these were certainly useful to know in order to care for and understand him more completely. However, we wondered if it might be helpful to have an area on the form for a synopsis of the assessment information — a patient profile. This would be especially useful to a nurse starting on the ward, or helping out for a day, to see at a glance the patient's major needs. At a suitable time in the day the nurse would then be able to take time to read through the assessment information and expand her knowledge of the patient, but the most important points would be highlighted in the assessment summary.

DIFFICULTY WITH ALs

As we have already mentioned, using the activities of living headings as a basis for assessment was something with which we were not familiar, and so we did indeed encounter some problems with this.

Our main difficulty was not in grasping the concept of ALs, as we had already used these to a certain extent in introducing the nursing process in the ward. Rather, the problem lay in the wording of the headings as given in *The Elements of Nursing*. These, we felt, were rather imprecise and open to various interpretations, thus creating difficulty in deciding which pieces of information were relevant to each heading.

For example, with John, pressure care became very important, and frequent and thorough assessment was required in this area. Unfortunately, one of us considered pressure care as being related to the AL 'maintaining a safe environment', whereas the other associated it with the AL of 'mobilising'. The ALs of 'eating and drinking' and 'eliminating' are also relevant in considering pressure area care. So, under which heading were we to record our information? This, however, was not our main concern. What did worry us as a result of this was the possibility that such important information as pressure area status could be missed altogether because the relevant information may be divided between several ALs and there is no specific indication of any one AL under which it should be assessed.

By referring to *The Elements of Nursing*, details of the type of information relevant to each heading may be obtained, but perhaps the inclusion of sub-headings on the form would help to clarify each AL, and make completion of the form a little simpler. The danger of omitting some problems might then be reduced, and consistency of patient care be maintained.

Concluding comments

In conclusion, then, we found this study both interesting and stimulating, although several problems did arise in the course of its completion.

These difficulties were mainly encountered in the practical application of the model in the ward setting. Although the framework seemed relatively easy to grasp, documentation in a concise and logical manner proved to be more difficult.

This does not appear to be unique to this particular model, and the question then arises of the practical application of the nursing process in general — can it become a practical proposition for everyday use in the wards, or will it be used merely as a learning exercise?

It would be unfair to attempt to answer that question on the basis of this project alone, especially as this particular model was only applied to one patient. However, in applying the nursing process to the care of other patients in the ward, albeit with a slightly different method of recording data from that shown here, we feel that patient care has improved. Although the approach is still relatively new and we are still adapating documentation to meet the needs of the ward, the nurses working on the ward now seem to have a greater understanding of the patients in their care, and their needs in all aspects of daily living. Continuity of care appears to have improved, and time is now used more effectively and efficiently.

It was perhaps because we had begun to settle into our own way of assessing patients, using headings similar to only some ALs (with more specific sub-headings) that we found the headings in this model rather vague. However, in general, we find that the concept of ALs encourages a more thoughtful and thorough approach to the patient, seeing him as an individual with many needs and problems, not all necessarily directly related to his disease condition.

It would appear, then, that although variations may occur in methods of documenting the stages of the nursing process, the concept of the process itself must surely be a basis for a more thoughtful approach to nursing, diverting it away from being task-orientated to being patient-centred by planning care according to his needs and problems which have been identified following systematic assessment.

This model provides a framework for such assessment. Although we experienced difficulty with it, and were especially concerned by the fact that some important information may be missed in using it, we felt that it did encourage comprehensive assessment, and to that extent could be a useful tool for both teaching and using, with adaptation, in the ward setting.

BIBLIOGRAPHY

Crow J 1977 The nursing process 1, 2, 3. Nursing Times 73: June 16. 23, 30
Hunt J M, Marks-Maran D F 1980 Nursing care plans. H M & M Publishers, Aylesbury
Kratz C 1979 The nursing process. Bailliere Tindall, London
Nursing Times Publication 1981 The nursing process. Macmillan Journals, Basingstoke
Nursing Times Booklet (supplement) 1978 Rediscovering the patient. Macmillan Journals, Basingstoke

9

A study in a psychiatric ward
using the model for nursing

Niall Grant and Bernard White

The nursing process in psychiatry

In implementing the nursing process in the care of patients, the nurse is involved in four separate but interdependent component stages: assessment of the patient, planning nursing intervention, implementing the planned care, and evaluating the success or otherwise of the plan.

Although the application of the nursing process can be seen to be quite straightforward in certain instances, some would say it is much more difficult to apply in psychiatry. A patient admitted to a general hospital with a chest infection is fairly easy to assess, and his nursing care straightforward to plan. Any progress he makes towards a return to health is easy to identify and to monitor. But what of the patient admitted to a psychiatric hospital for the treatment of an anxiety psychoneurosis? Here, application of the nursing process would seem to be less clear cut; the assessment itself would need to be carried out over a long period of time, and the nursing care plan would evolve slowly as more experience was gained of the patient's responses to his environment and to such treatment components as group therapy. Our contention is, however, that even in instances such as this, an attempt to plan realistic nursing care can only result in a more caring, comprehensive and consistent approach to the patient's needs by all his nurses, and this can only be to his benefit.

In studying our patient, we have looked at the value of the activities of living in helping us to assess her needs and plan her care. From the outset, one major advantage of the framework became clear. We found that not only were we trying to assess what the patient needed help in doing for herself, and what the problems were that were posed by her condition, but we were also looking very hard at what she *could* do independently. This made us very aware of our need to preserve her independence and therefore self-esteem; in a quite severely handicapped patient, this is of paramount importance.

THE PATIENT

Mrs McLeod was transferred to the ward for assessment of her organic brain syndrome. A lady of 86 years, she had been under the care of the hospital for the previous three years during which she had been attending the day hospital for elderly patients. She lived in sheltered housing, but her condition was now giving rise to anxiety, and it was decided to admit her for a full inpatient assessment. She was in fact admitted to another ward as an emergency for four days to await the availability of a bed in the assessment ward.

THE WARD

Mrs McLeod was admitted to a 22-bedded mixed assessment ward for elderly people with organic brain syndrome; the ward's function is to assess the extent of organic impairment, its cause and its treatment.

The ward was constructed in a basic T shape with bedrooms off the main corridor and a dining room/living room area at the end of the corridor. The layout proved easy for observation and appeared to lessen the chances of disorientation to place as most daytime activities were carried out in one area.

The ward was not purpose-built and did not easily meet the patients' needs for privacy in the larger bedrooms, toilets and bathrooms. However an attempt had been made to adapt the ward for the convenience of physically handicapped patients by the provision of wide doors and hand rails, but space was severely restricted in bathroom areas especially where wheelchairs and walking aids were needed by patients. The ward also lacked a small quiet area for patients who desired peace and quiet away from the often unsettling atmosphere of the living room with its television and record player, so disturbing to those who wanted/needed quiet.

The ward had a purpose-built kitchen where occupational therapy staff carried out any necessary cooking and safety-in-the-kitchen assessments. Other activities of living were assessed by both nursing and occupational therapy staff. A wide range of yet other assessments were carried out to estimate the extent of memory impairment and concentration, so the nursing staff were familiar with at least one phase of the process of nursing! There were planned activities to alleviate boredom and to cater for the patients' religious beliefs. Relatives were encouraged to visit and to help with the patients' assessments by providing useful personal history of the patient.

THE PROJECT

While the hospital and ward is accurately identified, all dates and personal details of the patient have been changed. Verbal permission to proceed with the project was obtained from the patient, her daughter, the physician superintendent, and the nursing officer of the unit.

The patient was studied for a fortnight during her admission, the purpose being to study the usefulness of the Roper, Logan and Tierney model for nursing in a psychiatric ward. What follows is therefore not a complete nursing care study from admission to discharge but is more a descriptive account of using and developing documents.

Application of the model for nursing

From the outset, one major advantage of using the patient assessment form became clear: we found that not only were we trying to assess what Mrs McLeod could not do in relation to each activity of living, but we were also looking very hard at what she could do independently.

We had initial anxieties about where our assessment of the patient's psychiatric state would 'fit' into the activities of living. Previously we had looked at such things as, for example, memory, orientation, thinking and perception. But these are psychological functions and are rightly associated with communicating. We also initially wondered where we could 'fit' such findings as delusions, disorientation and hallucinations. However, once we accepted that such findings would not fit naturally under just one AL, but would appear under several headings in different contexts, such problems became easier to deal with. For example, notes of Mrs McLeod's disorientation for time and place were relevant under both 'maintaining a safe environment' (she could wander off and become lost) and 'communicating' (she was occasionally unaware of her surroundings and our identity).

USE OF THE PATIENT ASSESSMENT FORM

The Patient Assessment Form as it appears in both *The Elements of Nursing* and *Learning to Use The Process of Nursing*

has space for recording biographical and health data on the left side, and AL data on the right. However, after assessing Mrs McLeod's dependence/independence in her activities of living on three separate occasions, we realised that the biographical and health data did not change so we decided to think of the biographical and health data as a separate document (Fig. 9.1, p. 120).

This permitted us to think along the lines of a two-page document with the AL data and the identified problems on the left page, and the nursing intervention which was agreed shortly after admission (Fig. 9.2, pp. 122-125) on the right. This enabled us to ensure Mrs McLeod's immediate safety, and to continue her established medication and dietary programmes, until such time as we could find out more about her. The data collected at the second assessment are shown in Figure 9.3 (pp. 126-129).

NURSING PLAN

Our records complemented rather than replaced the established ward records; progress notes continued to be entered in the standard nursing Kardex thrice daily as for other patients. The psychogeriatric dependency rating sheet (Fig. 9.4, p. 130) was filled in and it was considered to be an informative document, so much so that even late on in the project we felt that it would have to be an 'extra' document for a psychiatric patient. However, one of the editors asked us to think about it within an AL framework so with much prompting and thinking we realised that the information on the rating sheet could be documented under the ALs as shown on page 119.

We found that nursing staff showed considerable interest in our parallel records and they were used by the nursing team to plan Mrs McLeod's programme, and by all members of the team at the case conference to discuss her future.

Conclusion

The framework for nursing provided by the activities of living was found to complement procedures already in use in the hospital, and it was found to enhance the availability of knowledge about the patient and her progress.

More work needs to be done on the structure of the forms, in particular the Patient Assessment Form needs expanding to provide enough space for details to be clearly entered. From this exercise we suggest that the provision of a 'nursing plan' book or loose-leaf folder for each patient would be useful if this system were to be adopted by a ward. Nurses could enter their assessment of the patient on the left-hand page under AL headings; and goals, nursing intervention and evaluation could

Activity of Living: Psychogeriatric Dependency Rating Sheet

AL	Main Heading	Sections within heading	Information about patient
Communicating	Orientation	All sections	
	Behaviour	All sections	
	Physical	Hearing	
		Visual	
		Speech	
	Special physical disabilities	—	Blind in left eye
Breathing	Special physical disabilities	—	Breathless on exertion
Eating and drinking	Physical	Personal hygiene	
		Feeding	
Eliminating	Physical	Personal hygiene	
		Requires toileting	
		Urine — day	
		Urine — night	
		Faeces — day	
		Faeces — night	
Personal cleansing and dressing	Physical	Dressing	
		Personal hygiene	
		Oral	
		Washes	
		Cleans	
		Hair	
		Bath entry	
Mobilising	Physical	Mobility	
	Special physical disabilities	—	Needs Zimmer walking aid

be entered on the right-hand page thus this double-page document would be a comprehensive nursing plan. The document would be an ongoing record and one which any nurse starting work on the ward could refer to.

We were sufficiently impressed with the potential of the model to suggest that further studies should be undertaken, possibly using a group of patients, but certainly in a wide variety of clinical settings within a psychiatric hospital.

Figures to this chapter start on page 120.

Patient Assessment Form

Date of admission 29/9   Date of assessment 29/9

Surname McLeod   Forenames Mary Murdock

Male ☐   Age ☐ 86   Single/Married/Widowed ✓   Prefers to be addressed as
Female ✓   Other   Mrs McLeod

Date of birth

Address of usual residence   46/9 Bramwell House
                                    Tel: 943 1335

Type of accommodation   Sheltered housing for the elderly

Family/Others at this residence   nil

Next of kin   Name Mrs. Gwen McLaren   Address 16 Manton Crescent

                     Relationship Daughter   Tel. no. 887 5636

Significant others   Relatives/Dependents Warden of Bramwell House

                            Helpers   Home help 3 days a week

                            Visitors   none

Occupation   never had full-time employment.

Religious beliefs and relevant practices   none

Patient's perception of current health status   Walking and memory difficulties

Reason for admission/referral   Full assessment. Transferred from Ward B: admitted there from day
                                       hospital, pending availability of bed.

Medical diagnosis   Alzheimer - type dementia. Osteoarthritis. Right bundle branch block. Low-
                           grade urinary tract infection. Allergic response to ampicillin.

Past medical history   Dementia last 3 years. Requiring more supervision at night - nocturnal wanderi
                              several recent falls. Pacemaker 1977. Soluble aspirin. Frusemide. Arthritis L. hip and
                              L. eye injury 1974. L. simple mastectomy 1972, carcinoma.

Allergies   Ampicillin   Significant life crises Admission to hospital 4 days

Fig. 9.1 Patient Assessment Form: biographical and health data

Assessment of Activities of Living

AL	Usual routines: what he/she can and cannot do independently	Date Patient's problems (actual/potential) (p)= potential
● Maintaining a safe environment		
● Communicating		
● Breathing		
● Eating and drinking		
● Eliminating		
● Personal cleansing and dressing		
● Controlling body temperature		
● Mobilising		
● Working and playing		
● Expressing sexuality		
● Sleeping		
● Dying		

Assessment of Activities of Living

Date 29/9

AL	Usual routines· what he/she can and cannot do independently	Patient's problems (actual/potential) (p) = potential
• maintaining a safe environment	Walks with aid of walking frame Cannot hear or see very well Becomes confused towards evening	Unsteady on feet Poor sight ℞ eye No sight Ⓛ eye Hard of hearing Disorientated for time and place Poor short term memory Possible urinary tract infection Skin rash — possible allergy to ampicillin Implanted cardiac pacemaker
• communicating	Verbal communication clear Evidence of confusion at nights Sight/hearing deficits Quickly becomes irritable	Anxiety Disorientation increased by new environment Misidentifies people at night
• Breathing		Breathless on exertion
• Eating and drinking	Enjoys food Can feed herself Takes fluids well	Slightly obese
• Eliminating	Can manage toilet and handwashing with minimum assistance	Becomes breathless on exertion Possible urinary tract infection Isolated episodes of loose stools reported last two days (possible drug reaction) Urinary incontinence at night Disorientation
• Personal cleansing and dressing	Can manage well given time Cannot manage big bath	

Fig. 9.2.1 Patient Assessment Form: AL data on admission

Nursing Intervention

Goal

Evaluation

Supervise walking with frame meantime
Speak to her clearly and slowly – don't
shout
Observation room – height adjustable bed –
no bedside mat – check brakes on furniture
Commence 4 hourly TPR chart
Weigh
Midstream urine tomorrow
Careful observation in evening and
during night

Clear, verbal messages
memory and orientation jogs
Assess orientation and memory during
evening
No extensive questioning

Backrest in bed
Observe for breathing difficulties
during night
Observe extent of breathlessness
on walking

Assess appetite and fluid intake tonight

Chair in bathroom
Assess frequency of micturition and
incontinence
Record bowel actions
Supervise visits to bathroom

Assess abilities

Fig. 9.2.2 First nursing plan

Assessment of Activities of Living

Date 29/9

AL	Usual routines: what he/she can and cannot do independently	Patient's problems (actual/potential) (p) = potential
● Controlling body temperature		Slightly pyrexial
● mobilising	Will shuffle with walking frame	Unsteady on feet Falls reported Complains pain (L) knee (? arthritis)
● Working and playing	Enjoys conversation Cannot hear or see well	Cannot see IN or door labels Cannot hear IN/Radio Hears speech with difficulty Easily irritated
● Expressing sexuality	Looks clean and tidy Takes pride in personal appearance	Lack of privacy
● Sleeping	Reported to sleep well	Disorientation Urinary incontinence

Fig. 9.2.1 Patient Assessment Form: AL data on admission (contd)

Nursing Intervention

Goal   Evaluation

4 hourly TPR chart ;
soluble aspirin
Good fluid intake — hourly drinks
during day
Bedrest if feeling cold

Supervise walking with frame
Assist rising from bed
Soluble aspirin as charted
for pain
Check fit of slippers

To be assessed

Provide privacy where possible —
but discreet supervision / observation
always
Female staff meantime

As "breathing" and
"eliminating"
Comprehensive night report

Assessment of Activities of Living

Date 30/9

AL	Usual routines: what he/she can and cannot do independently	Patient's problems (actual/potential) (p) = potential
● maintaining a safe environment	Can concentrate only for short periods Good recall of past life events Correctly orientated during morning and afternoon	Easily trips and staggers on feet Unsteady rising from chair Right bundle branch block – no "blackouts" since pacemaker inserted Finds walking frame a "damn nuisance" – refused to use it occasionally Memory of day's events fragmentary Irritable on questioning and with other patients Severe disorientation with time and place during evening
● Communicating	Speaks clearly and responds appropriately during day – not at night Appropriate non-verbal and emotional backup Enjoys reminiscing Expresses needs clearly Looks suspicious and frightened at night Occasional verbal outbursts of verbal aggression (? catastrophic reaction) "Go boil your head" (to doctor) Identifies people correctly during day – not at night Remembers names, not at night Relaxes happily with daughter at visiting Expresses anxiety about shadows at night	Sensory deficits Diurnal variation in orientation Poor concentration Poor short-term memory Perception threshold increase at night – illusions
● Breathing	Breathes easily and quietly at rest No cough. Does not smoke Breathless after 15 minutes on feet	Walking excursions not possible Needs rest in bathroom and occupational room
● Eating and drinking	No particular likes and dislikes Food and fluids taken well	Can she prepare food for herself ?
● Eliminating	Manages in toilet Needs assistance in getting there Pays careful attention to hygiene	Urinary incontinence single episode last night No more diarrhoea
● Personal cleansing and dressing	Can dress herself given time Help needed with tights, shoes, zips Hygiene assistance as above Has special brassière – ① breast prosthesis prefers to manage this garment herself	Not completely independent Likes to dress herself and gets frustrated when help required Embarrassed about mastectomy and breast prosthesis

Fig. 9.3.1 Patient Assessment Form: AL data on second assessment

Nursing Intervention

Goal		Evaluation
Prevention of accident to self and others	Close observation especially in evenings Intervene when irritation shows Speak at eye level – touch Use name – prefers "Mrs. McLeod" Memory and orientation jogs Change activity or environment if concentration/interest fails Try walking steps without frame – 2 nurses, short distances only High chair in sitting room	No accident
Improved quality of life	Memory and orientation jogs Speak clearly and slowly at eye level Frequent, short conversations Assess likes and dislikes Minimise shadows at night	Evaluate weekly
Minimal breathlessness	Continue TPR chart Wheelchair for visits outside ward Monitor length of time on feet at any one time	
Independent eating and drinking	No restriction on diet Hourly drinks Occupational room for assessment of kitchen work	
Normal elimination Minimal embarrassment	Encourage her to go to toilet regularly Record all episodes of incontinence	
Contented with pride in appearance	Try Ambulift for big bath Female staff assistance in bathroom Use own toiletries – daughter will replenish stocks Personal clothing being washed Daughter will take all laundry Any soiled articles to be washed quickly in ward first Needs hospital hairdresser appointment Cleans own teeth – dentures Chiropodist to visit	

Fig. 9.3.2 Second nursing plan

Assessment of Activities of Living

Date 30/9

AL	Usual routines: what he/she can and cannot do independently	Patient's problems (actual/potential) (p) = potential
● Controlling body temperature	Dresses appropriately Comments on high temperature in ward and asks for better ventilation	Slight pyrexia continues
● Mobilising	As first assessment plus: cannot negotiate steps or stairs adjusts own position frequently in bed and in chair – all pressure areas healthy	Bumps into low tables in her path Becomes very anxious when walking supported only by nurses Will not take good steps – shuffles only
● Working and playing	Enjoys knitting for short periods if help is given with pattern	Did not enjoy the morning's music and movement session – felt isolated as she could not see and hear well
● Expressing sexuality	Takes pride in her personal appearance Uses toiletries Speaks warmly and with dignity about her marriage	Conscious of restricted privacy in hospital Embarrassed at mastectomy and breast prosthesis
● Sleeping	Slept soundly last night, waking only following single episode of incontinence Settled for the night more easily than expected	Embarrassed and ashamed of incontinence
● Dying	States she's "a grand old age" Does not express anxiety to leave hospital Appears quite content while correctly orientated	

Fig. 9.3.1   Patient Assessment Form: AL data on second assessment (contd)

Nursing Intervention

Goal		Evaluation
Normal IPR	As first assessment	
Increased independence	As first assessment plus: appointment with physiotherapist for walking education Persist with aided walking meantime	
Prevention of boredom	For further occupational therapy assessment Appointments made for optician and E/N I physician	
Comfortable with her femininity	Preserve bedroom/bathroom privacy — but observation always Compliments on appearance Female staff assistance only for dressing and bathroom	
Rested on wakening	Manages adjustable height bed well No cotsides No draw sheets/inco pads Try two pillows instead of backrest Soluble aspirin before retiring Record frequency of incontinence	
	Daughter to visit tonight — Sister will give her an opportunity to discuss her mother's future Don't cut her off if she speaks of death, let her talk about it	

Fig. 9.3.2 Second nursing plan (contd)

PSYCHOGERIATRIC DEPENDENCY RATING SHEET

Name: _Mrs. Mary McLeod_   Age: _86 y/o_   Unit No: _12345_

Assessed by: _M. Grant_   Designation: _SIN_   Ward/~~Dept~~: _A_   Date: _6/10_

1. ORIENTATION

Yes	No	
✓		Name in full
	✓	Age (years)
✓		Relatives — Recognise
✓		Relatives — Name
✓		Staff — Recognise
	✓	Staff — Name
	✓	Bedroom
	✓	Dining Room
	✓	Bathroom
	✓	Belongings

2. BEHAVIOUR

N	O	F	
	✓		Disruptive
✓			Manipulative
		✓	Wandering
✓			Socially Objectionable
	✓		Demanding Interaction
		✓	Communication
	✓		Noisy
✓			Active Aggression
	✓		Passive Aggression
	✓		Verbal Aggression
	✓		Restless
✓			Destructive — Self
✓			Destructive — Property
✓			Affect — Elated
✓			Delusions/Hallucinations
			Speech Content

N = Never
O = Occasionally = 2/5 days or less
F = Frequently = 3/5 days or more

3. PHYSICAL

HEARING

	Full
	Slight
✓	Severe
	Deaf

VISUAL

	Full
✓	Slight
	Severe
	Blind

SPEECH

✓	Full
	Slight
	Severe
	Dumb

MOBILITY

	Full
	Stairs
✓	Aids
	Assistance
	Chairfast
	Bedfast

DRESSING

	Full
✓	Verbal
	Partial
	Assistance

PERSONAL HYGIENE

Verbal Guidance		Physical Assistance
✓	Oral	
✓	Washes	
✓	Cleans	
✓	Hair	
	Bath entry	✓

N	O	F	
			REQUIRES TOILETING
		✓	URINE—DAY
		✓	URINE—NIGHT
		✓	FAECES—DAY
		✓	FAECES—NIGHT
✓			FEEDING

SPECIAL PHYSICAL DISABILITIES (SPECIFY)

Needs zimmer walking aid
Blind in (L) eye.
Breathless on exertion.

NB.   ANSWER ALL QUESTIONS — ADD FREE COMMENT OVERPAGE IF DESIRED.

Fig. 9.4 Psychogeriatric dependency rating scale (form already in use in ward)

10

A study of a patient at home

using the model for nursing

Mary Cooke and Sheila Moir

Introduction

It was with some trepidation, yet a marked degree of enthusiasm that we contemplated the project with which we had become involved. The first and most obvious requirement was for both participants to become totally familiar with the theoretical framework we were setting out to evaluate, that is, the model for nursing comprising the activities of living and the nursing process as described by Roper, Logan and Tierney in *The Elements of Nursing*. The lecturer was conversant with the mode of thinking called the nursing process but the district nurse was not, and neither had used the model.

After reading *The Elements of Nursing* we decided to set objectives for ourselves to enable a critical appraisal to be made at the conclusion of the project and these are listed below:

- to test the appropriateness of the proposed assessment form for community nursing use
- to estimate the usefulness or otherwise (in a community setting) of the proposed model for nursing
- to incorporate the process of nursing when using the proposed model
- to judge patient benefit in terms of improved patient care, as a direct result of using the model for nursing
- to obtain the opinions of the undernoted participants involved in using the model for nursing, namely the district nursing sister, the patient and relatives, district nursing colleagues, and the nursing officer.

The patient who was to play such a vital part in the programme was carefully sought, with the intention of involving the caring relatives in some measure, without whom care in the community would often be impossible. Throughout the four-week duration of the study the patient was attended by one of the authors, the district nurse, relieved on days off by one colleague only, and she most willingly contributed her opinions about the project.

Perhaps one of the most thought-provoking areas of the

study was in relation to the use of suitable documentation. Some of the questions uppermost in our minds were:

- what should the documentation consist of?
- in what form should it be produced?
- in what way might the nursing plan be modified?
- would the documentation be useful to other members of the primary health care team?

Throughout the study, apart from the essential documentation, copious notes were taken of impressions gained thus providing a ready reference which proved of inestimable value when seeking to create an interesting and informative account of the project.

In the remainder of the chapter we will attempt to demonstrate step by step the sequence of events which led eventually to the appended conclusions.

The patient and her family

THE PATIENT

Mrs Martin was a 41-year-old woman who lived at home with her husband Andrew and two daughters — Mary aged 16 and 15-year-old Fiona. Mrs Martin had been a fit and active woman until a year ago when she became ill with what was thought to be bronchitis. She took self-prescribed medication for some time before finally attending her general practitioner by which time she was suffering quite severe pain. Following several hospital investigations it was discovered that Mrs Martin had a large tumour of the lung which was found to·be inoperable. Mrs Martin and her family were informed that she was suffering from cancer and that it would be necessary to commence cytotoxic therapy as soon as possible.

When first referred to the District Nursing service, Mrs Martin had just completed a fourth course of cytotoxic therapy, and on meeting her it was obvious that she was a very frail, weak and debilitated person weighing only 32 kg. Not surprisingly Mrs Martin's appetite was poor mainly because of the nausea which so commonly accompanies cytotoxic therapy. Another major concern involved difficulty with bowel movements and rectal pain caused by the presence of haemorrhoids: the constipation was sufficiently severe for the patient to require frequent oral aperients and enemata. She was aware of the fact that she was suffering from cancer and understandably this led to bouts of deep depression.

THE FAMILY

Until the time that the district nurse commenced visiting it was evident that Mrs Martin had been very well cared for at home by her husband and daughters Fiona and Mary. Although Mr Martin worked full-time as a store manager and also had part-time employment for three evenings per week in a local public house, he always ensured that his wife was 'left comfortable'. He helped her to wash herself each morning before he went to work and assisted her into an immersion bath every evening before settling her in bed. It was Mrs Martin's wish that her family care for her as much as possible. She was aware of her condition, but her husband did not want her to be informed of her very poor prognosis. Mr Martin was fully aware of his wife's illness and prognosis and, although initially shocked and upset, reacted very courageously, his main aim being to keep their home life as near to normal as possible. For this reason, they refused the offer of a homehelp.

Fiona and Mary were both informed about their mother's condition and both proved to be of great help in caring for her and carrying out household tasks. Both girls were very diligent and progressing well at school. Mary appeared to accept her mother's illness quite well, but Fiona was very reluctant to discuss the illness with anyone. She seemed to understand the circumstances, but could not accept the fact that her mother was dying. Her father was very helpful and often discussed the situation with her.

Mrs Martin's sister-in-law, who worked as a cleaner in a nearby school, visited for one hour each morning and two hours each afternoon. While there she helped with the preparation of meals and household tasks. Several neighbours also visited to help with shopping and one in particular visited frequently. This meant that the patient was rarely alone in the house, thus helping to prevent the feeling of depression that so often occurred when she was alone.

The family appeared to function harmoniously within the cultural norms and organisation of the society to which they belong.

HOME CIRCUMSTANCES

The Martins lived in a three-apartment council flat. It was situated in deck-access housing in a fairly busy city suburb area. The flat was modern with excellent cooking, washing and toilet facilities and always appeared to be clean. Although Mrs Martin's bedroom was small, there was sufficient room to manoeuvre; an adequate working surface being available at the bed-side when carrying out nursing procedures and cupboard space available for the storage of materials and equipment. The patient was warm and comfortable while in bed and several pillows were provided, as the possibility of breathing problems was always present. Because of her emaciated condition, bed-clothes were left to hang quite loose. The bathroom with a modern suite, was conveniently situated next to the bedroom, enabling Mrs Martin to walk to the toilet unaided, a degree of independence she valued. Heating was provided by electric storage heaters and although these are often criticised for causing a dry atmosphere, no such problems were identified in this instance as Mrs Martin had no cough or sputum.

INTRODUCING THE FAMILY TO THE PROJECT

When the patient and her family were visited for the first time they were given information about the proposed project. From an ethical point of view, it was agreed that Mrs Martin would be asked if she and her family would be willing to participate. Mrs Martin's permission was obtained, indeed she was very willing and was pleased with the thought that she might be helping to improve standards of care given to other patients.

While the patient assessment was being carried out, the family were encouraged to contribute and it was fascinating how they seemed to understand so quickly the type of information required. At this stage they were also introduced to the Nursing Plan which it was agreed would be left in the home, and ways in which they could help to ensure continuity of care were discussed. The family greatly appreciated being involved in the discussions regarding the care of their wife/mother and volunteered to maintain records. Because of their enthusiasm, they were provided with the second Roper, Logan and Tierney book *Learning to Use the Process of Nursing* (1981). They read the book with much interest and said it helped them to understand more clearly the aims of the present project.

The nursing study

A great deal of thinking was done by the two authors before starting the study and as mentioned in the introduction, the major difficulty was planning the documentation which eventually was kept in a specific sequence in a folder. We will now describe some of our difficulties.

PATIENT ASSESSMENT FORM: BIOGRAPHICAL AND HEALTH DATA

Because of the complex nature of caring for patients in their own homes, plus the fact that caring is often shared by a variety of carers, professional and otherwise, we realised that the suggested headings on the Patient Assessment Form: biographical and health data, had some omissions. We therefore made some minor amendments to the form and added other items which are essential information for the community nurse. For use in the community we would also want to alter the spacing. The following comments relate to the Patient Assessment Form: biographical and health data (Fig. 10.1, p. 138):

Type of accommodation
Under this heading we suggest a large enough space to record information on two other aspects:

deficiencies which may concern the building itself, e.g., dampness, or the living situation, e.g., overcrowding. Either of these circumstances may greatly affect the patient's health status and would require attention

entry to the house. This information is of crucial importance when a number of nurses are visiting a patient, e.g., the nurse may be in possession of a key; a key may hang on a string behind the letterbox; or it may be that the door is left unlocked.

Significant others
We suggest that this heading would require a reasonable space to permit a description of the care context within which the patient is found, that is the 'others' who are involved in caring apart from professionals, e.g., relatives who live with the patient; relatives/friends who visit routinely and are involved in giving care of some nature; neighbours who may be involved; the homehelp and so on.

Family's perception of patient's health status
Because of total family involvement it is necessary to be aware of the above, particularly when coping with terminal illness at home. Preparation of relatives prior to bereavement necessitates an awareness on the part of the nurse about the degree of perception the family possess, regarding the patient's terminal state. This information could go under 'Patient's perception of current health status'.

Past medical history
A larger space may be required particularly for patients with a long history of chronic illness as one so often finds in district nursing.

General practitioner
The name of the patient's general practitioner, his surgery address and telephone number is essential. It would also be beneficial to have his home address and telephone number should they be required.

Hospital consultant
The name and hospital address of the consultant in charge of the patient is required.

There were other pieces of information which must be recorded when nursing a patient at home and we put them following the PAF: assessment of ALs (Figs 10.3 and 10.4) on Figures 10.5-10.7 as follows:

Medications
A large area for prescribed medications is needed. And separately, a note of medications taken by the patient — not prescribed by the doctor (Fig. 10.5, p. 152).

Treatments
A similar area is required for recording treatments (Fig. 10.5).

Appointments
It is necessaty to record future appointments arranged, e.g., a return to the outpatient department to see the consultant, including details of transport arrangements (Fig. 10.6, p. 153).

Equipment on loan
In the community, patients receive a loan of equipment of various kinds from a variety of sources such as hospital equipment; equipment borrowed from voluntary organisations, e.g., WRVS, British Red Cross Society; health board equipment. It is essential to record details of such equipment to ensure its safe keeping and its return when no longer required by the patient (Fig. 10.6).

Supportive services
Apart from nursing and medical services, others of a statutory or voluntary nature are frequently contacted to assist in the total care of patients and their relatives. Part of the form is required for the inclusion of these points in the overall plan of care (Fig. 10.6).

Record of visits
When visiting in the home, it is imperative to keep a calendar record of visits (Fig. 10.7, p. 154).

Initially we felt it essential to have as a heading *Description of Patient*, providing for the relief nurse scanning the documentation, a concise picture of the patient whom she has not yet met. However, as we became familiar with the model, we realised that the model itself should provide an overall picture of the patient and his problems, thus eliminating the need for anything else by way of description. We did however want a description of what we called the *Immediate Nursing Environment*. Details regarding the suitability/unsuitability of the area in which nursing is being given is beneficial to all members of the nursing team, particularly relief nurses who may be visiting the patient for the first time. Sometimes it is necessary to make minor alterations to the patient's room for his benefit or the benefit of caring relatives or both for example, placing meaningful objects on the affected side of the patient who has had a stroke to encourage him to use the disabled side of his body; or perhaps the provision of adequate space to enable walking practice for the patient in a room which was previously cluttered with furniture. We put this description at the end of the twelve ALs on Fig. 10.4.1 (pp. 146-147).

Initially too we thought it would be necessary to have a separate heading *Economic Factors* with details about the patient's financial circumstances where appropriate; these facts may indicate if further assistance is required particularly from the Department of Health and Social Security. Concern about finance can often retard recovery and require the attention of the district nurse. We decided however, that these details could go under the AL of working (and playing).

Similarly it was felt that provision would have to be made on Figure 10.1 (p. 138), for details regarding *Facilities* within the patient's home, those which have a direct bearing upon his ability to be independent or otherwise, namely bathroom facilities, cooking facilities, laundry facilities and the method of heating the home. Because of the close association between these facilities and the activities of living however, we decided to consider each under the appropriate activity when assessing the patient initially:

toilet facilities considered under *Eliminating*
bathing facilities considered under *Cleansing and Dressing*
cooking facilities considered under *Eating and Drinking*
heating the home considered under *Controlling Body Temperature*

It may be assumed by some that assessment of any activity of living should only be made if there are problems in relation to that activity, requiring the attention of the nursing team. It is important, however, in relation to the facilities mentioned above, that the information be recorded whether or not there is a problem, thus providing essential information regarding the home in which the patient lives. This is of value to the relief visiting nurse who is not familiar with the patient.

Furthermore, should there be, for example, an electricity strike in winter, it would be very simple to determine by consulting the documentation belonging to each patient, those patients at risk to hypothermia, so enabling intervention to be planned at an early stage in the emergency situation.

PATIENT ASSESSMENT FORM: ASSESSMENT OF ACTIVITIES OF LIVING

To provide easy reference when speaking with the patient and family about activities of living, a decision was made to devise a checklist (Fig. 10.2, p. 139) consisting of a series of 'triggers' to the memory under each activity of living, and appropriate in particular to patients being cared for at home. Indeed these 'triggers' are consistent with the AL diagram at the end of the twelve chapters in *The Elements of Nursing*. The rationale behind the decision evolved from the realisation that the use of any model for nursing initially presents something of a challenge to nursing personnel, whether qualified or student

nurse, essentially because of the completely new approach to patient assessment. The checklist is recognised to be incomplete itself, merely suggesting some of the factors most commonly considered in relation to each activity of living.

While still in our preliminary stage of planning how to document the activities of living we noted certain points which could cause confusion and could be difficult when using this model. As we anticipated these possibilities in relation to Mrs Martin's future care, we record them for interest.

Pressure areas
The decision to assess pressure areas under the activity of mobilising was made, because of the close association between immobility and the development of pressure sores. Consideration was also given to recording it under:

the activity of eliminating, incontinence being one of the main predisposing factors to the development of pressure sores
the activity of personal cleansing and dressing which relates to the care of the skin, as it is the tissues and skin over the bony prominences which are constantly under review with regard to the same problem
the activity of eating and drinking, because of the fact that poor nutrition renders the tissues vulnerable to the development of pressure sores.

It is highly possible that registered nurses (who may not refer to a checklist such as ours, but simply use the headings as a guide) may decide to assess pressure areas under any of these categories. This could lead to confusion among junior members of staff in particular.

Spiritual needs
Although it is recognised that religious practices may affect many of the activities of living in a variety of ways, it was decided to place the spiritual needs of the patient under the activity of dying, because of the possibility that during the terminal stages of an illness (as was the case with this patient) perhaps more than at any other stage of life, the patient may express some need for guidance or comfort of a spiritual nature.

Pain
The assessment of the patient in pain could be problematic when using the model. Should the pain experienced be in relation to eating and drinking, eliminating, mobilising or dying, it could be assessed in relation to the appropriate activity. Should the patient's pain, however, consist of, for example, severe headache; angina at rest; pain in the abdomen not related to eliminating; there is no appropriate 'activity' to facilitate assessment of such. Furthermore, the assessment of this subjective and lonely experience requires a very detailed assessment before nursing intervention can be planned to the patient's benefit, and before the total description of such would be meaningful to a nurse who might be visiting for the

first time. A space for this kind of information we decided, would have to be provided on the form.*

Other

There was indecision about the appropriate place for recording pulse rate and blood pressure; recording of levels of consciousness should the patient become comatose (as might have been the case with Mrs Martin); and the recording of certain skin/tissue conditions, e.g. jaundice, skin eruptions, and oedema, which were complications Mrs Martin might encounter.*

When actually using the model for the first assessment, the format even with the help of our checklist was thought to be rather laborious and time-consuming. However, this problem was really due to the fact that the approach was new and we were not knowledgeable about its use. In fact despite the difficulties already mentioned, the model was of great benefit when carrying out the initial assessment, and even more so for subsequent assessments.

It had several advantages:

- it became easier to assess the patient, both physically and mentally and there was less risk of missing problems
- actual and potential problems were identified clearly
- it was possible to plan care more fully due to the thorough initial assessment
- the format of the assessment gave a much clearer picture of the patient
- nursing colleagues had more information available
to them prior to visiting the patient for the first time.

Advantages such as these can only lead to an improvement in standards of nursing.

NURSING PLAN

The Nursing Plan we devised for community use, consisted of the model for nursing with sections developed opposite each activity of living to accommodate assessment; actual/potential problems; short-term goals, intervention; and evaluation (ALs 1-6 on Fig. 10.3.1, pp. 140-141 and ALs 7-12 on Fig. 10.4.1, pp. 146-147).

A modified version of the Plan as already mentioned, was left in the patient's home along with a flow chart for noting the patient's daily progress. This Plan included the patient's problems, but only the actual problems were recorded in the home; as Mrs Martin was not aware of her poor prognosis, it was decided that potential problems would not be listed. The Plan was used by all caring relatives; they were able to check the problems, the patient's goal in relation to these and the nursing intervention required. This meant that Mrs Martin

*In retrospect, and referring again to *The Elements of Nursing* we realise that pain would go under 'Communicating', coma would go under 'Sleeping', skin and tissue conditions would go under 'Personal cleansing and dressing'. But at the time, we did not immediately see them categorised under such ALs.

was well cared for during 24 hours each day, by either nurses or relatives. The family enjoyed using the Plan, entering notes on the flow chart, supplying information about care given to Mrs Martin, medication administered, pain level experienced and her general condition at various times of the day. They all felt very involved in her care and appreciated having the opportunity to participate in this way.

The main Nursing Plan was kept at the District Nurse Centre and when subsequent assessments were made, continuation sheets were placed over the original data, but maintaining the original headings along with the activities of living (ALs 1-6 on Figs 10.3.1, 10.3.2 and 10.3.3, and ALs 7-12 on Figs 10.4.1, 10.4.2 and 10.4.3). Each continuation sheet was dated and numbered as reassessment was carried out. Using this method it was simple to read about the patient's progress right through to the initial assessment, and goals not achieved were quickly noted.

As we indicated earlier, we would probably want to re-design the documents and for general use, for example, the space taken by Figs 10.5-10.7 (pp. 152-154) could be much reduced. But certainly our folder contained all the information required by the district nurse.

Opinions about the use of the model

DISTRICT NURSES

We discussed the model and process of nursing with several district nurses in the area. First opinions regarding use of the model consisted of the usual comments 'We do not need any more changes'; 'The system is fine in its present form'; and 'This would be far too time-consuming'. However with more information and the help of the checklist they decided that the use of these twelve activities of living would really be very beneficial when carrying out patient assessments. They agreed that use of the model for nursing would provide a clearer picture of the patient, the family and the home situation.

Part-time nurses were very enthusiastic about this form of patient assessment as it gave them a great deal more information. They found this particularly helpful as, at the moment, patient records are not readily available to them. The relief nurse who took over the care of Mrs Martin for a few days, said that she felt she knew the patient very well before she ever met her because the assessments were so precise. It was considered that this must surely prove beneficial to the patient as well as to the nurses concerned.

The general mood, therefore, was one of enthusiasm. However, there are still some nurses who do not wish to change from the present format.

PATIENT AND RELATIVES

Mrs Martin was astonished that the relief nurse had so much information concerning her circumstances when the nurse visited for the first time. Mrs Martin felt relieved that the nurse did not have to ask her any more questions, explaining that when staff visited previously, before use of the model, they seemed to take more time becoming familiar with her problems, treatment and goals.

The family stated that they were more aware of the patient's problems and thus felt more able to help. They were grateful to be involved in caring for their relative and appreciated sharing some of the responsibility. All members of the family were genuinely interested in the model and felt that Mrs Martin was very well cared for.

NURSING OFFICER

The nursing officer was of the opinion that use of the model would be of benefit to her because it would enable her to quickly glean more concise information regarding the patient's problems. She considered that the eliciting of potential problems in relation to each activity is highly desirable, as the documentation currently used in her area does not require any statement of such so there is no way of acknowledging and emphasising the need for 'prevention' of problems. The information provided would also assist her by demonstrating the needs of patients and relatives, particularly when assessing the total circumstances, for example, prior to mobilising the night nursing service.

She also thought that this method had enormous potential as a teaching tool helping not only student district nurses to learn about nursing in the community, but also assisting students taking the basic programme for registration when they accompany the district nurse as observers.

Conclusions

Having completed the project, it is hard to envisage the use of a problem-solving approach to patient care without incorporating for the purpose of patient assessment, a model for nursing. It would seem essential to decide upon a model to provide a theoretical framework which would facilitate assessment of the patient in total.

In our interpretation of the model and the process of nursing, an attempt was made to provide a format that would enable the whole cycle to be documented in such a way, that the reader could see at a glance the following sequence of events:

Assessment of ALs → Statement of problems →
Short-term goals → Intervention → Evaluation

The process of nursing is in itself merely a methodical and logical way of thinking, which can be applied to any decision-making procedure. In itself it is inanimate; it is the use of a model for nursing that gives it purpose and meaning. The model and the process then, go hand in glove. It seems incredible — and we criticise ourselves — that some experienced nurses are only now realising the necessity of approaching patient care in such a logical fashion.

This model for nursing proved to be very effective when used to assess this patient, terminally ill, in her own home. Perhaps this was due to the fact that the patient had a variety of problems, both actual and potential, in relation to most activities of living. The model served the purpose of focusing the attention of the assessing nurse in relation to each activity of living, thus enabling problems to be elicited in a thorough and methodical way so preventing certain problems from being missed.

Difficulties were encountered, however, with certain nursing observations which could legitimately fit into more than one activity of living, but perhaps these uncertainties would be eliminated as one became more familiar with using the model for nursing. For some observations however, no place could readily be found and perhaps some additional 'spaces' should be added to the 12 ALs to allow for the recording of such material.

Another inadequacy, as far as community use is concerned, was the biographical data part of the Patient Assessment Form as suggested by Roper, Logan and Tierney. This is chiefly because of the complex nature of caring for patients and their families within the context of home in contradistinction to hospital. Nursing in the home setting involves a variety of carers whose skills will vary from professional to novice and the utilisation of a wide range of resources, both material and financial. Recording of these components, among others, is vital if continuity of care is to be meaningful and if information is to be shared with other members of the primary health care team.

On evaluation of the patient's response to nursing intervention it was decided that the patient did benefit from use of the model by the assessing nurse largely because actual and potential problems were readily elicited, thus enabling appropriate action to be taken to assist the patient to prevent or cope with her problems.

Consultation with those colleagues and relatives who had been either directly or indirectly involved in patient care confirmed the fact that the use of the model for nursing with the process of nursing, provided for each a sense of satisfaction.

Reviewing our conclusions, we considered we had met the objectives formulated at the outset of the project.

Projections for the future

In recent years, a number of models for nursing have been posited. Some are rather complicated as models and attempting to apply them to the practice of nursing requires a considerable amount of imagination. The Roper, Logan and Tierney model for nursing certainly has a semblance of simplicity; one can immediately identify with commonly occurring activities such as eating and drinking, communicating, mobilising, or sleeping. Using it as a framework along with the so-called process of nursing as a mode of thinking does work in practice as we have shown, but a major area of concern is the recording of the data concisely yet adequately. We consider that, with practice, this could be performed with considerable speed and accuracy. For use in the community too, we have suggested that provision should be made on the form for some extra details related to significant others, and related to the home environment.

Even if this model with the process of nursing were not used always by qualified nursing staff, we see it as a particularly helpful tool for the use of students. Though time-consuming to think through and use this approach (and it would be so on the first occasion) a consideration of the physical, emotional, socio-cultural, and economic aspects (where relevant) of each AL, and the use of this information when assessing, planning, implementing and evaluating patient care would encourage a logical approach to the practice of nursing which hopefully would perseverate when the period of studentship had been completed.

The model could be used as a teaching tool to demonstrate to *student nurses* on community secondment, the method of assessing patients within their own homes. Should the format already be familiar to them in the hospital setting, they would readily identify with it, providing them with an exercise in transfer of learning. Other students who require an insight into district nursing, for example, *health visitor students* and *general practitioner trainees*, could be assisted to learn in a similar manner.

Registered nurses, desiring to become involved in district nursing following an acceptable period of post basic experience would find the transition from hospital to community somewhat easier should the approach to patient assessment be a similar one. *Student district nurses* could be introduced to the model during the theoretical component of the course, allowing them opportunity to make the application of theory to practice throughout the practical placements. Provision of suitable documentation for student use would be essential, should it not be available in the area where practical experience was being gained. Updating courses for all qualified nurses would, therefore, be necessary to familiarise them with the model, special attention being given to practical work teachers, to enable them to give the necessary support to students under their supervision.

Should the decision be made to transfer nursing records with the patient upon admission to hospital, the information made available to hospital colleagues would surely be of great value, and facilitate continuity of care to the benefit of the patient. Apart from encouraging improved standards of patient care, generally speaking, an analysis of the records used in such a model for nursing would assist in adding to that body of knowledge, which is *nursing* — so essential for any 'research-based profession' as was indicated in the Report of the Committee on Nursing (Briggs Report, 1972).

Figures to this chapter start on page 138.

Patient Assessment Form

Date of admission	Date of assessment 21 Sept.

Surname **Martin**   Forenames **Catherine**

Male ☐	Age **41**	~~Single~~/Married/~~Widowed~~	Prefers to be addressed as
Female ✓		Other	**Mrs Martin**
	Date of birth		

Address of usual residence *Flat 2/20 30 Main Street.*

Type of accommodation *Deck - access 3 apartment council flat with bathroom.*
(incl. mode of entry) *Excellent cooking, washing and toilet facilities.*
Key in district nursing centre.

Family/Others at this residence *Husband and two daughters (aged 16, 15)*

Next of kin   Name *Andrew Martin*   Address *As above*

Relationship *Husband*   Tel. no. —

Significant others Relatives/Dependents *Husband, 2 daughters (Mary 16, Fiona 15)*
Sister - in - law Mrs Craig; works nearby; visits 1 hour am, 2 hours p—

Helpers

Visitors *Family, friends*
neighbours Mrs. MacRae and Mrs. Wood and Mrs. Roy.

Occupation *School cleaner*

Religious beliefs and relevant practices *Roman Catholic*

Perception of current health status
Patient *Knows she has cancer*
Family *Husband and daughters know she has poor prognosis*

Reason for referral *Home nursing required. Referred by GP*

Medical diagnosis *Ca. of lung. Weight loss, poor appetite; haemorrhoids, constipation.*

Past medical history *Was fit and active till 9/12 ago.*

GP address, phone: *Dr. Alan Brown*   *5 Hillview Road*   *Home: 10 Cedar Avenue*
surgery and home   *068 6789*   *0746 - 473*

Allergies | **Significant life crisis**

Fig. 10.1 Patient Assessment Form: biographical and health data (modified version of Roper, Logan and Tierney form)

ACTIVITIES OF LIVING CHECKLIST

Maintaining a safe environment	Communicating	Breathing	Eating and drinking
Hazards	Vision	Character	Facilities
Cleanliness	Hearing	Cough	Dentition
Storage of medicines	Speech	Sputum	Independence
Sensory deficit	Non-verbal	Dyspnoea	Diet type
Other	Mental state	Cyanosis	Diet adequacy
	Pain	Pain	Daily fluid intake
	Other	Smoking habits	Dislikes
		Other	Pain
			Other

Eliminating	Personal cleansing and dressing	Controlling body temperature	Mobilising
Facilities	Facilities	Heating system	Independence
Independence	Independence	Personal clothing	Aids in use
Bowel habits	Interest	Bedclothes	Muscle tone
Bladder habits	Cleansing aids	Exercise	Joint mobility
Incontinence	Dressing aids	Other	Pain
Abnormal elimination	Other		Pressure areas
Pain or discomfort			Other
Other			

Working and playing	Expressing sexuality	Sleeping	Dying
Income status	Self image	Hours of sleep	Knowledge
Occupation	Self worth	Rest periods	Acceptance
Recreation	Self projection	Difficulties	Family
Independence	Sexual difficulties	Aids to sleeping	Spiritual needs
Other	Other	Other	Pain
			Other

Fig. 10.2 'Trigger' or checklist for assessing ALs

AL	Assessment ①	Date 21 Sept.
maintaining a safe environment	Home surroundings good. Unsteady gait but wishes to remain independ⟨ent⟩ Can walk from bed to toilet safely but requires help on stairs Medicines kept in locked cupboard and supervised by husband	
Communicating	Speech normal; communicates well. Hearing good. Wears spectacles for reading Enjoys company and prefers to have opportunity to discuss illness Tends to become depressed if alone; worries about outcome of treatmen⟨t⟩	
Breathing	No dyspnoea at present; tended to be breathless prior to cytotoxic therap⟨y⟩ Intermittent cough but no sputum Smokes 10-12 cigarettes daily Often complains of chest discomfort but no specific pain	
Eating and drinking	Modern kitchen facilities; electric cooker Able to feed self but appetite poor; mainly fluid diet. Well-fitting dent⟨ures⟩ Currently often nauseated; Maxolon prescribed Daughter enjoys cooking & encourages mother to eat	
Eliminating	Modern toilet facilities near bedroom Able to go to toilet unaided Urinary output adequate; continent; no dysuria Often constipated; takes oral Dulcolax tab 2 nocte & frequently require⟨s⟩ a Microlax enema	
Personal cleansing and dressing	Modern bathroom facilities; no shower Able to wash self each morning; basin at bedside Helped into bath by husband every evening Family eager to assist Skin/pressure areas intact	

Fig. 10.3.1 Patient Assessment Form: assessment of ALs 1–6 with associated problems, goals, intervention and evaluation

Problems	Short-term goals	Intervention	Evaluation
• Unsteady gait : at risk of falling.	Reduced anxiety Optimum independence	Education of family to help patient maintain safe environment. Assistance with stairs and exercises.	3 Oct. Able to walk short distance unaided : up and down stairs with help.
• Tendency to depression • (p) may become more depressed & dependent as condition deteriorates	Improved mental state	Support. Discuss problems. Help to communicate freely.	1 Oct. Able to talk freely to nurses and family about cancer
• Carcinoma of lung • (p) likely to become breathless → distress	Allayed anxiety Eased discomfort	Monitor respirations. Health education re smoking, breathing, exercises. Teach patient to expectorate.	3 Oct. Breathing now more relaxed No dyspnoea
• Poor appetite: emaciated, (wt. 32 kg) • (p) mouth may become dry & coated • (p) pressure sores	Adequate dietary intake Mouth free from infection Healthy skin & tissues	Education of patient & family re nourishing foods (Complan). Protect from kitchen smells. Teach to use mouth wash.	3 Oct. Now able to tolerate light diet & fluids Nausea continues but not so severe
• (p) Haemorrhoids, constipation • (p) incontinence • (p) pressure sores	Relieved discomfort Improved bowel motion	Dulcolax tab. 2 nocte. Enemata as required. Proctosedyl cream to haemorrhoids.	28 Sept. Moderate relief to haemorrhoids Less constipated
• Unable to bathe without assistance • (p) pressure sores	Optimum independence Healthy skin & tissues	Education of family re care. Supervision of care.	1 Oct. Seems comfortable Skin intact Family coping well

AL	Assessment ②	Date 5 Oct.
Maintaining a safe environment	Continues to have unsteady gait ; condition now worse due to pain in both legs Drugs still supervised by husband House clean & tidy	
Communicating	Now speaks openly about cancer ; needs chance to alleviate anxi Easy to talk to Tendency to depression continues	
Breathing	No further breathlessness Still smokes ; now 15 – 20 cigarettes daily Has had intermittent chest pain ; no undue anxiety	
Eating and drinking	Appetite improving ; now tolerates more solid foods ; less nausea Had oral infection (thrush) but now cleared so appetite better Weight gain of 4.4 kg	
Eliminating	Still manages to toilet unaided Slight dysuria ; improving Bowel habit changed from constipation to diarrhoea & sometimes incontinent	
Personal cleansing and dressing	Help only for bathing Pressure areas intact	

Fig. 10.3.2 Patient Assessment Form: second assessment of ALs 1–6 with associated problems, goals, intervention and evaluation

Problems	Short-term goals	Intervention	Evaluation
		Teach patient passive exercises to prevent contractures	5 Oct Still requires help on stairs
		Continue to give support; this seems to have helped	
	Controlled pain		5 Oct. Breathing relaxed & seems normal
• Remains very thin • (p) pressure sores	Continued nourishing diet Mouth free from infection Healthy skin & tissues		10 Oct. Feeling better Eating light meals Pressure areas healthy
• Diarrhoea with incontinence	Normal bowel function	Microlax enema given Provision of incontinence pads	13 Oct. Spurious diarrhoea due to faecal impaction Satisfactory result to enema
		Situation monitored daily	10 Oct. Skin intact

AL	Assessment ③	Date 15 [
maintaining a safe environment		
Communicating	Good relationship with patient Able to discuss anxieties freely	
Breathing	No further breathlessness Still smoking Occasional pain (R) side on exertion ; relieved by analgesic	
Eating and drinking	Appetite deteriorated again due to bowel problems ; patient anxio No sickness Mouth clean & moist No weight gain	
Eliminating	Large faecal impaction ; fear of suppositories / enemata due to painful haemorrhoids ; not much relief from analgesic creams Some incontinence No further dysuria	
Personal cleansing and dressing	Requires more frequent cleansing because of incontinence Very conscious of personal cleansing	

Fig. 10.3.3 Patient Assessment Form: third assessment of ALs 1–6 with associated problems, goals, intervention and evaluation

Problems	Short-term goals	Intervention	Evaluation
			Good relationship
• Pain ⒧ side	Controlled pain	Continue breathing exercises Pethidine 100 mg or MST 1 tab. 1 PRN for severe pain	18 Oct. Less pain but still some discomfort
	Diet with high fibre content to stimulate bowel action	Educate family re high fibre diet	20 Oct Has taken small meals with family
• Faecal impaction with overflow diarrhoea • Painful haemorrhoids • (p) further incontinence	Improve bowel habit Alleviate pain (haemorrhoids)	Dulcolax suppositories 2 with good result Procte sedyl cream to haemorrhoids	10 Oct Less pain from haemorrhoids Still prone to constipation

AL	Assessment ①	Date 21 Sep
Controlling body temperature	Electric storage heaters, electric fire in sitting room Temperature adequate, comfortable surroundings, bedclothes sufficien Patient's temperature 36.5°C	
Mobilising	Can walk slowly. Muscle tone quite good, but thin and weak Independence encouraged but poor prognosis → bedfast Up to sit some evenings with family	
Working and playing	Worked as school cleaner till present illness Husband has steady work plus part-time job Receiving Mobility Allowance & awaiting receipt of Attendance Allow Advice given re tax rebate Interests include knitting, media & family	
Expressing sexuality	Alopecia due to cytotoxic therapy; wears wig although uncomfortabl Very conscious of appearance Good relationship with husband; very "caring"	
Sleeping	Sedation of Halcion tab. 2 Often awake at night with generalised aches & pains; relieved by o Pethidine 100 mg	
Dying	Not aware of poor prognosis: husband and daughters told life expectancy is 3–6 months. Family seem prepared but will need sup Priest visits on regular basis	
Immediate nursing environment	Patient nursed in small, modern bedroom Sufficient work surfaces & storage space for nursing facilities Bedroom next to bathroom so goes to toilet unaided Room warm. Bedclothes sufficient.	

Fig. 10.4.1 Patient Assessment Form: assessment of ALs 7–12 with associated problems, goals, intervention and evaluation

Problems	Short-term goals	Intervention	Evaluation
• Enforced bedrest • (p) pressure sores	Increased time out of bed Healthy skin and tissues	Family helping patient Teaching patient simple leg exercises Teaching family re prevention of pressure sores Provision of sheepskin rug and heel muffs	29 Sept. Progressing slowly with exercises Up to sit in evenings
• Depressed when alone in house • (p) severe depression	Fewer episodes of depression	Family, friends, neighbours advised to visit at different times Encourage hobbies Nurse to visit when patient alone Involve patient in care plan	4 Oct. Friends helpful Patient resumed interest in knitting
• Alopecia; very self-conscious • (p) loss of feminin-ity	Preserved femininity	Help with personal appearance Listen to problems	4 Oct. Able to discuss problems
• Unable to sleep without sedation	Restful undisturbed sleep	Halcion tab. 2 & Pethidine 100 mg to settle at night	4 Oct. Not sleeping well; lies awake worrying about illness Refuses change of sedation
• Poor prognosis • (p) fear of dying and death	Freedom from anxiety	Listen to patient Listen & discuss with husband & daughters especially younger daughter	4 Oct. Husband & older girl coping well but still unable to discuss with younger daughter

AL	Assessment ②	Date 5 ᴜ
Controlling body temperature	Body temperature has remained normal	
Mobilising	Still able to walk to toilet unaided but needs help on stairs Feels better because appetite better Up to sit with family each evening Generally more mobile	
Working and playing	Taking more interest in knitting	
Expressing sexuality	Still self-conscious about alopecia ; hopes hair will grow in before Christmas	
Sleeping		
Dying		

Fig. 10.4.2   Patient Assessment Form: second assessment of ALs 7–12 with associated problems, goals, intervention and evaluation

Problems	Short-term goals	Intervention	Evaluation
		Encouraged to go up & down stairs with help	10 Oct. Up to sit in lounge each evening
		Encouraged with hobby	10 Oct. more involved with family and friends Arms sore when knitting

AL	Assessment ③	Date 15 Oct
Controlling body temperature		
Mobilising	Spending longer periods in bed due to weakness caused by persistent constipation/diarrhoea Able to walk up + down stairs a few days ago but feels too weak to attempt it now	
Working and playing	Appears to have lost interest in hobbies; depression due to constipation/ diarrhoea since completion of cytotoxic therapy Friends visit when patient feels well enough	
Expressing sexuality	Depressed recently but still very conscious of appearance	
Sleeping	Sleep disturbed by pain caused by haemorrhoids; relieved by c Pethidine 100 mg & Ativan 2 mg	
Dying	On several occasions voiced concern re dying Family do not wish her to know of poor prognosis	

Fig. 10.4.3 Patient Assessment Form: third assessment of ALs 7–12 with associated problems, goals, intervention and evaluation

Problems	Short-term goals	Intervention	Evaluation
• Prolonged bedrest can only walk short distance • (↑) muscle wasting	Up to sit with family Improved muscle tone	Teach passive limb exercises	20 Oct. Able again to walk up & down stairs under supervision of husband
• Depressed	Regained interest in surroundings	Encourage family & friends to discuss hobbies/topics of interest	18 Oct Feels better Up to sit with family
• Depressed	Preserved self-image & self-worth	Encourage daughters to interest mother	20 Oct. Daughters helpful; great asset to mother
• Sleep disturbed by pain	Undisturbed sleep	Halcion tab. 2 & Pethidine 100 mg as night sedation Analgesic cream to haemorrhoids	20 Oct. Not sleeping well but does not wish sedation changed
• Anxiety about condition but unaware of poor prognosis	Reduced anxiety	Support patient Support family esp. younger girl Spiritual support from priest : visits regularly	20 Oct. Patient more calm

Medication Prescribed

Date	Prescription	Dose	Route	Frequency	Discontinued
21 Sept.	Pethidine	100mg	oral	4-6 hourly	
	Ativan	1mg	oral	3 times a day	
	Distalgesic	2 tab.	oral	as required (outwith times for Pethidine)	
	Halcion	2 tab.	oral	night sedation	
23 Sept	m S T - 1	1 tab.	oral	as required for severe pain or at night with sedation	

Non-Prescribed Medication Taken by Patient

Treatment Prescribed

Date	Prescription	Frequency	Response	Discontinued
1 July	Proctofoam to haemorrhoids	as required	part effective	
	Enemata bucrolax	as required	effective	
	Noratex cream to pressure areas	3-4 times per day	effective	
24 Sept.	Nystan oral suspension	4 times per day	successful treatment of oral thrush infection	6 Oct.
	Dulcolax suppositories 2	as required	effective	
	Proctesedyl haemorrhoid cream	as required	part effective	

Fig. 10.5 Medication and treatment prescribed

Equipment on Loan

Date	Article	Source		Returned
23 Sept.	Sheepskin rug Sheepskin heel pads	District nurse centre District nurse centre		

Appointments

Date	Place	Reason	Conveyance	Arranged

Supportive Services

Service	Date	Remarks	Discontinued
Social worker			
Meals on wheels			
Home help			
Marie Curie Foundation			
Twilight/night nursing			
Physiotherapy			
Occupational therapy			
Speech therapy			
Chiropody			
Day hospital			
Voluntary services			
Other			

Fig. 10.6 Equipment on loan, appointments and supportive services

Record of Visits

Year	1	2	3	4	5	6	7	8	9	10	11	12	13	14	15	16	17	18	19	20	21	22	23	24	25	26	27	28	29	30	31
January																															
February																															
March																															
April																															
May																															
June																															
July																															
August																															
September																					≡	—	≡	≡	—				—	—	
October	—	—			—	—	—	—	—			≡	≡	—	—	—			—		≡		—				—				
November																															
December																															

Fig. 10.7 Record of visits to home

11

A study in a neurosurgical ward
using the model for nursing

Marjorie Armstrong and Anne Jarvie

Good nursing (for those who are sick) consists simply in observing things which are common to all sick, and those which are particular to each sick individual.

Florence Nightingale, 1861

The nursing process:
the stage we were at

When we agreed to write this chapter, we knew little about the Roper, Logan and Tierney model for nursing but were not starting from scratch in our thinking about the nursing process. In the neurosurgical unit, we had been discussing and using the nursing process for about ten months. From a review of the literature it would seem that for some nurses who introduce the nursing process mode of thinking, one of the benefits is a concomitant change from a task orientation method of organising nursing to patient assignment. This was not so in our case. Patient assignment had been the ward practice for several years. Nevertheless, as a staff, we had been dissatisfied with its results.

As a Senior Nursing Officer with an interest in the neurosurgical unit (and with a remit for the implementation of research findings) and as a sister of one of the wards, we had been very much involved in the discussions throughout the ten month period when the staff were re-thinking about nursing itself and how it was planned, carried out and evaluated in the unit. Using a trial, discussion and amendment method the staff eventually devised an assessment form and it required that we introduce a nursing plan format. Looking back on these ten months we believe that the overall quality of care had improved in that each patient was now viewed as a whole person, not just a diseased part of a whole person. The most difficult part had been the evaluative phase. We had to admit that, in the past, much useful information especially

information about the effectiveness of nursing had been committed to memory rather than to paper, and finding a suitable way to document data had been and still was a particularly thorny problem.

The ten months of effort had altered our thinking and approach but it had also resulted in some much more overt changes. Changes had been made in ward routine for example, sleeping and resting were now viewed as a vitally important area for consideration when planning nursing. The patients were now wakened by the day staff at 7.45 a.m. and the ward was darkened between 1–2 p.m. to allow patients to rest. Also the routine report session from night staff to day staff was omitted although important and relevant details were passed on to the nurse in charge. The nurses working in teams went straight to the patients to whom they were assigned and used the nursing plan to guide their activities. This change in routine had turned the nursing plan into a working tool and had been instrumental in proving the usefulness of such a tool.

The nurses gathered after lunch for 'the report' which had now taken on a new dimension. Two-way communication occurred, each team reporting on and discussing patients with the other nurses present. The nurses felt more confident now that they were in possession of much more information about the patients and were involved in planning their nursing. They particularly liked the emphasis now given to the patients' social and psychological state and well-being. They seemed to be more aware of their responsibility to and for their patients and hopefully saw this as a measure of their accountability. As for the learners, they felt slightly overawed initially when attending these 'reports' but soon appreciated the advantages, both to the patients and themselves, of this kind of reporting session. Some were even heard to comment that they dreaded going to a ward where this kind of reporting was not practised. Opportunity was given to learners to write the report on their patients and this was much appreciated as nurses have been guilty in the past of not 'teaching' the art of report writing.

This re-thinking of the nursing plans and the use of the nursing process was therefore already in progress when we were invited to participate in the project using the Roper, Logan and Tierney model for nursing which incorporates the nursing process. However, although both contributors had been using the process mode of thinking for ten months and had been involved in introducing changes which they consider improved the nursing in the unit, neither had actually used the model for nursing.

Choosing the patient

We were asked to try to choose an adult, male patient who had been admitted to the unit because of a head injury and it was with great care that we chose John.

After an evening spent in a public house, John returned to his mother's house only to discover that he had no key. Following unsuccessful attempts to waken his mother, he attempted to climb the drain pipe to gain entry through a window. Unfortunately, two flights up, John lost his grip and fell to the ground. After ten days in the Intensive Therapy Unit, John was transferred to our neurosurgical ward, which is bright, well equipped and built in the race-track design. This mixed ward has 23 beds divided into single and four-bedded rooms, John being in one of the latter. He spent 15 days in our care, before being returned to his referring hospital and although his consciousness level had improved he was still greatly dependent for most activities.

John was unconscious on admission so we decided to do two admission assessments of his ALs. On one we recorded his status as we interpreted it from our observations (Fig. 11.2, pp. 160-161). On the other (Fig. 11.5, p. 164) we attempted to acquire from his brother and sister a profile of John as he had been before the accident occurred, though both acknowledged the limitations of this information as John had lived alone for quite some time. We hoped that as the patient recovered consciousness, this second assessment would help us to orient John in relation to his customary activities and assist in his recovery.

We considered our position ethically with regard to using information about John in our project particularly in view of the fact that on admission John was unconscious. It was decided to discuss this matter with John's family who were most interested in what we were doing and readily gave permission to use any material that would be helpful to us.

A model for nursing: how it worked for us

The model for nursing based on the activities of living as described by Roper, Logan and Tierney certainly proved a useful aid to help us to conceptualise what nursing is all about. This did not come easily; much reading and discussion was necessary before we were able to work with this particular way of thinking. But we considered that understanding the process of nursing became more real while using the activities of living as the basis of patient data collection in order to make an assessment. The assessment form that had previously been devised for use in the ward in which our study was to take place had incorporated some of the activities of living, so perhaps we experienced fewer difficulties in this area than others may. However terminology such as 'expressing sexuality' did cause some concern. Frequent referral to the chapter on this activity in *The Elements of Nursing* was necessary before sufficient confidence was established to allow questions and prompts to flow naturally when discussing this activity. Potential problems in discussing and recording both this activity and also that of dying could be envisaged if it were decided to introduce this Patient Assessment Form for general use in the ward.

We felt also that more guidance was needed for us to feel confident in applying the evaluation phase of the process using this model. However, we were certainly forced to think long and hard about this phase, for which we are grateful. Consideration had to be given to the frequency with which evaluation should take place, how success or failure of the implementation phase could be measured and how this information was to be documented. Being keen to move away from the traditional Kardex for progress notes towards individual patient's nursing notes stored in separate folders further complicated our thinking on documentation. Although this phase did not come easily we have become more acutely aware of the need to recognise actual and potential problems. The fact that a resolved 'actual' problem becomes a 'potential' problem hit us like a bolt from the blue.

Overall, however, the positive approach that emerges towards planning nursing when applying this model and this way of thinking to each individual patient appeals enormously.

Before illustrating our use of the documents with data collected about John it is necessary to make some comments about the documentation. When John was admitted we assessed him and his circumstances using the Patient Assessment Form (PAF) suggested in *The Elements of Nursing*. We refer to the left-hand side as PAF; biographical and health data (Fig. 11.1, p. 159) and this did not prove difficult to use; adequate space was provided for all the details we considered necessary to record about John. The right-hand side we refer to as PAF: assessment of ALs (Fig. 11.2, pp. 160-161) and this was found to be most acceptable. It was a useful framework within which to think about an individual patient and the nursing he is going to require, and the twelve ALs used seem to incorporate all the possible needs of an individual. However, some thought was required when marrying certain problems with the appropriate AL. For example, the potential problem — development of pressure sores — will in many cases fit in with 'personal cleansing' or 'eliminating' but seemed to us to be more closely related to 'mobilising' in view of John's immobility due to unconsciousness.

Another concern was the time, effort and material used in recording. When considering the documentation required to reflect the nursing process, one of the criticisms frequently levelled is that more time has to be spent on report writing. With this in mind we were anxious to use all documents at our disposal in such a way as to avoid unnecessary writing. We therefore made three decisions:

- to extend the right-hand side of the PAF: assessment of ALs to include the associated 'goals' and 'evaluation' (Fig. 11.2, p. 161).
- to document the implementation phase of the nursing process on a separate sheet as nursing plan; intervention (Fig. 11.3, p. 162) rather than as a column betwen 'goals' and 'evaluation' because we wanted it to be kept at the bedside. Leaving the nursing plan at the bedside helps the nurses, particularly the learners, to realise that nursing requires to be prescribed just as medicines are prescribed. It also means that the nurses listen more attentively and become more involved in reporting sessions when relieved of the need to write down details of care required by each patient as the report is being given.
- to record observations such as temperature, pulse, respiration, and conscious level on the charts currently used in the unit, the TPR chart and the Glasgow Coma Scale (Fig. 11.4, p. 163), and not on the above forms.

We had only a limited time during this project to think through, devise and use the documentation. With more time to test the use of the model incorporating the process of nursing, it is possible that we would experiment further and change some of the documents.

The reactions of others

STUDENTS ON THE INTENSIVE CARE COURSE

As a facet of our teaching/learning we decided to ask the students undertaking the Intensive Care Course in our hospital to use these forms as part of an assignment.

A teaching session on the model for nursing incorporating the nursing process preceded the distribution of the forms. The immediate reaction was that it would not work in a highly specialised unit. The Patient Assessment Forms were initially unacceptable to them; the students felt threatened by the questions that they imagined would be required to elicit the necessary information. Their particular worries were associated with the terms 'significant life crises' and 'expressing sexuality'. However, following further discussions each student agreed to do a nursing study using the forms provided. The reporting back session proved most interesting.

The Patient Assessment Forms were found to be a useful and helpful method of collecting information. All agreed that they had learned much more than usual about their patient and had therefore been better able to support and care for both the patient and the family. The two areas described above as their particular areas of worry did not present them with the problems they had anticipated. The students stated that they could see real potential for this way of thinking about nursing and also the use of these forms in intensive care situations. While accepting that these students, who were undertaking a course, do not prove the usefulness of such a way of thinking, working and documenting in the everyday real life situation, it was nonetheless interesting and encouraging to note the difference in their attitudes before and after being introduced to the model for nursing.

WARD STAFF

The nursing staff working in the ward in which our nursing study took place found it interesting to hear about the project in which sister was involved. As they had already been thinking about the patient as an individual for some time and practising team nursing they felt that they would be able to adapt fairly readily to the activity of living mode of thinking and the documentation necessary to reflect this thinking.

OTHER NURSES

Some members of our profession, however, support a view that was expressed at a meeting recently — the profession is going overboard about the nursing process and no matter what argument one puts forward it is an indisputable fact that disease is what brings the patient into care and so disease, not health, will always be the starting point in our thinking. It was further suggested that it is unrealistic to expect nurses to think of a patient as a whole person who happens to have a diseased part. This point of view seems to highlight the real need for education or perhaps re-education? It would seem that many in our profession are firmly entrenched in a 'disease' model for nursing and have little concept of assisting the patient and family to maintain health or prevent disease or learn to cope with disability.

Conclusions and recommendations

This exercise has been stimulating, interesting and well worthwhile. It has made us study in depth another approach, indeed in our opinion a better approach, in providing a framework within which to use the nursing process. The model, as described in *The Elements of Nursing,* where the patient has a life-span from conception to death during which he experiences changes in his activities of living, and can manifest changes in these activities along the dependence/independence continuum, seems a reasonable approach to take.

However, one should not underestimate the amount of time and effort that would be required should a decision be taken to promote a model for nursing as a useful framework for individualised patient care. Teaching and discussion on a regular basis would be absolutely essential; each member of staff, senior and junior, being given the opportunity to attend. It would be pointless to introduce new learners to this approach and then allocate them to practical situations where staff did not understand the re-orientation in thinking. This is not to say that existing care is unacceptable but the activities of living model has so much more potential and is conducive to assisting both patient and family to appreciate the need for self-care.

While working on this project we have become convinced that a nurse should be appointed with a remit for the implementation of the nursing process, preferably using the model for nursing as a framework. This person would require to be 'bursting with enthusiasm' for successful implementation to occur. Communication with and among staff is extremely difficult nowadays, especially with the shorter working week, and the success or failure of this mode of thinking being adopted seems to us to be inextricably linked with good communication.

Having seen the effect that the term 'nursing process' has on people it seems appropriate to suggest that very careful consideration be given to all terms used to describe a model for nursing and the activities of living. Bias once formed is so difficult to erase.

Much thought has been given to possible alternative terms for 'expressing sexuality' and 'significant life crises' but we find ourselves unable to make any suggestion. We now consider that careful definition of these terms would perhaps be sufficient, because we experienced less difficulty the more we familiarised ourselves with the model and the appropriate chapter on the activity in *The Elements of Nursing.*

Dying is another subject that we have tended to shy away from in the past, but attitudes are in the process of changing and the need for open discussion on this subject is now recognised. It is to be hoped that by retaining this activity on an Assessment of Activities of Living Form, senior staff will continue to be reminded of their responsibility to support all ward staff, and learners in particular, when they actually experience caring for a dying patient and are confronted with death itself; hopefully too, nurses will become more aware of the needs of a dying patient and his/her family. Collaboration between tutorial staff, ward staff and nurse managers is essential if nurses are ever going to come to terms with their remit with regard to the dying patient.

While accepting that the model for nursing incorporating the nursing process has much to offer, we consider it necessary to advocate flexibility if routinisation of forms is to be avoided. Those interested in trying this framework should continue to ask themselves questions such as 'do we need this framework for all patients in all situations?', 'do we need every phase and appropriate document for every patient?' We have continued to use the twelve activities of living as the framework for drawing up our nursing plan but we are not convinced that it is essential to have all twelve ALs on a standardised form. More and more we have come round to thinking that headings on a blank sheet of paper may be all that is necessary provided the nurse had had practice in using the AL framework. She would then identify only the ALs which were appropriate to consider for a particular patient and record only these on the blank sheets.

On re-reading our completed chapter we were struck by the frequency of use of the words 'document' and 'documentation' and considered if our readers might be justified in believing that we were only concerned with sheets of paper. We believe not, because it seems to us that from a legal point of view, we as a profession, are now absolutely compelled to think about documentation and if this can be achieved, while at the same time reflecting what nursing really means, so much the better.

We are exceedingly grateful for having been given the opportunity to test a model for nursing and hope our comments will be helpful to others.

atient Assessment Form

e of admission 29 Sept.

Date of assessment 29 Sept.

name Brown

Forenames John

le [✓]

Age 38

Single/Married/Widowed
Other Separated

Prefers to be addressed as
John

nale [ ]

Date of birth

dress of usual residence

10 Edinburgh Avenue.

e of accommodation

4 apartment flat

mily/Others at this residence none

xt of kin

Name Jane Brown

Address 7 Stirling Avenue

Relationship mother

Tel. no. 441 6362 (Sister : Elizabeth Green)

gnificant others

Relatives/Dependents 2 sisters, 1 brother.
Wife with whom he wishes to be reunited.

Helpers

Visitors Sister and brother. Wife (although separated) showed concern.

cupation Unemployed : made redundant 2 years ago.

ligious beliefs and relevant practices Catholic - no longer practising

tient's perception of current health status Unconscious on admission

ason for admission/referral Head injury - fell from drainpipe 2 flights up.

edical diagnosis Diffuse head injury
pelvis, clavicle, L) elbow, L) wrist.

ast medical history Alcoholic with cirrhosis of liver. Chronic bronchitis

llergies none known

Significant life crises Separation from wife 4 years ago

ig. 11.1 Patient Assessment Form: biographical and health data

Assessment of Activities of Living

Date 29 Sept.

AL	Usual routines: what he/she can and cannot do independently	Patient's problems (actual/potential) (p)= potential
● Maintaining a safe environment	Totally dependent Restless	● (p) may sustain injury when restless

● Communicating	Verbally : unable to speak
	Non - verbally : restless when apparently in pain
	    restless when requiring to
	    eliminate
		● Unable to make known most needs
		● (p) adverse reaction to environment when awareness returns

● Breathing	Cough reflex present ; dyspnoeic ; chest infection (known bronchitic) Haemothorax treated on admission to Intensive Therapy Unit : chest drain now removed. Wound site clean & intact on admission	● Dyspnoea ● chest infection/purulent sputum ● (p) infected wound site ● (p) obstructed airway
● Eating and drinking	Unable to be fed by oral route on admission Nasogastric tube passed and left in situ for feeding purposes	● (p) inadequate nutrition ● (p) difficulty maintaining gastric tube in situ (restless)
● Eliminating	Urinary catheter in situ on admission to ward Urethral discharge (not present prior to catheterisation) Incontinent of faeces	● Urethral discharge ● Incontinence of faeces ● (p) loss of bladder tone ● (p) constipation : impacted faeces
● Personal cleansing and dressing	Dependent for all care Hair - clean Skin - clean ; superficial abrasions no red areas/pressure sores Mouth - tongue coated & dry Eyes - "sticky"	● Skin abrasions ● "Dirty" mouth "sticky" eyes ● (p) Infected mouth, eyes, skin
● Controlling body temperature	Temperature elevated on admission : chest infection established as cause	● Perspiring
● Mobilising	(L) hemiparesis : confined to bed (L) arm : plaster of Paris Unable to change position independently but some movement when restless	● Dependent ● (p) pressure sores, contractions, deformities
● Working and playing	Unemployed	● (p) may be rendered unemployable as result of injury
● Expressing sexuality		
● Sleeping	Differentiate sleep/unconsciousness	● Coma
● Dying		● (p) death Relatives : poor/good understanding of seriousness of condition

Fig. 11.2 Patient Assessment Form: assessment of ALs and associated goals and evaluation

Goal	Nursing intervention	Evaluation
To keep the patient safe		Remained unharmed throughout his stay in the ward
To anticipate needs by careful observation To alleviate pain and assist with elimination		Patient appeared comfortable & therefore needs were thought to have been met No verbal response during stay in ward
To relieve dyspnoea To maintain clear airway To overcome chest infection To keep wound site (drain) free of infection		1 Oct. Breathing improved: oxygen therapy discontinued 13 Oct. Chest infection improved: physiotherapy, positioning, antibiotics 13 Oct. Wound remains clean & intact
To maintain adequate nutrition To establish oral feeding as soon as possible		Initial difficulty in absorption of feeds: adaptations made by dietitian 3 Oct. Commenced oral fluids: tolerated well 9 Oct. Semi - solid diet & fluids: tolerated well
To re-establish normal elimination patterns To alleviate discomfort from urethral discharge To keep clean & dry (incontinent)		13 Oct. Patient remained incontinent of faeces Uridome in situ on discharge 5 Oct. Urethral discharge cleared
To keep patient clean & dry To establish self- care as soon as possible To heal skin abrasions Clean & moist mouth Clean & dry eyes		Self-care not established 4 Oct. Mouth improving as oral fluids commenced 6 Oct. Eyes clean but preventive care continued 13 Oct. Skin abrasions improving slowly without treatment
To reduce temperature to normal To remove discomfort by bathing		2 Oct. No longer perspiring: temperature lower 13 Oct. Low grade pyrexia still evident
To establish independence in movement To keep skin intact & healthy		Gradually able to move all parts of body except (L) arm with help Despite effort, little progress in walking
To return to full awareness		Glasgow Coma Scale. Eye opening 4 Motor response 2 Verbal response 1
		Sister & brother accepted situation: shielded mother from gravity of situation

See Fig. 11.3

Nursing Intervention

AL	Date ordered	Prescription	Signature	Date discontinued
Maintaining a safe environment	29 Sept. 29 Sept. 29 Sept.	Use cot sides at all times Use geriatric chair with attached table when up Supervise at all times	J. Smith J. Smith J. Smith	
Communicating	29 Sept. 29 Sept.	Stimulate patient by verbal communication & by touch at each contact Analgesia as medically prescribed to relieve pain (indicated by restlessness)	J. Smith J. Smith	
Breathing	29 Sept. 29 Sept.	Oro-pharyngeal suction (usually by physiotherapist but as necessary by nurses) Oxygen therapy via humidifier	J. Smith J. Smith	7 Oct. 1 Oct.
Eating and drinking	29 Sept. 3 Oct. 5 Oct. 9 Oct.	Nasogastric feeding (as chart) bolus method 3 hourly Commence oral fluids Remove nasogastric tube Commence semi-solid diet & supplement with nourishing fluids	J. Smith J. Smith J. Smith J. Smith	5 Oct. 5 Oct.
Eliminating	29 Sept. 29 Sept. 5 Oct. 5 Oct. 5 Oct.	Catheter toilet 4 hourly Continuous catheter drainage Remove catheter : C.S.U. Uridome in situ : 4 hourly toilet Aperient as required	J. Smith J. Smith J. Smith	5 Oct. 5 Oct. 5 Oct.
Personal cleansing and dressing	29 Sept. 29 Sept. 29 Sept. 6 Oct. 6 Oct.	Bedbath X 2 am + pm Mouth toilet 4 hourly toothbrush/paste Bathe eyes with saline 4 hourly Bathe eyes am + pm Immersion bath (plaster in polythene bag)	J. Smith J. Smith J. Smith	5 Oct. 6 Oct.
Controlling body temperature	29 Sept. 29 Sept.	Tepid sponging as required Assess need for prescribed aspirin suppositories & give appropriately	J. Smith J. Smith	4 Oct.
Mobilising	29 Sept. 29 Sept. 5 Oct. 11 Oct.	Bed rest ; 2 hourly position change Elevate head of bed Up to sit for periods no more than 30 minutes Attempt ambulation with assistance of 2 nurses	J. Smith J. Smith J. Smith J. Smith	
Working and playing	29 Oct.	Stimulate as much as possible		
Sleeping	29 Oct.	Leave patient as comfortable as possible to allow rest between episodes of care		

Fig. 11.3 Nursing plan: intervention

	Eye opening *Score*	Motor response *Score*	Verbal response *Score*
high score		**6** If command such as 'lift up your hands' is obeyed	
		5 If purposeful movement to remove painful stimulus such as pressure over eyebrow	**5** If oriented to person, place and time
	4 If eyes open spontaneously to approach of nurse to bedside	**4** If finger withdrawn after application of painful stimulus to it	**4** If conversation confused
	3 If eyes open in response to speech	**3** If painful stimulation at finger tip flexes the elbow	**3** If inappropriate words are used
	2 If eyes open in response to pain at finger tip	**2** If the patient's arms are flexed and finger tip stimulation results in extension of elbow	**2** If only incomprehensible sounds are uttered
low score	**1** If eyes do not open in response to pain at finger tip	**1** If there is no detectable response to repeated and various stimuli	**1** If no verbal response

A normal person would score 15 on the scale; the lowest possible score is 3 which is compatible with, but does not necessarily indicate, brain death. A score of 7 is used as a definition of coma.

Fig. 11.4   Glasgow coma scale (form already in use in ward)

Assessment of Activities of Living

Date 29 Sept

Patient's problems
(actual/potential)
(p)= potential

AL	Usual routines: what he/she can and cannot do independently
● Maintaining a safe environment	Lives alone normally & looks after self On night of accident was intending to stay with mother
● Communicating	No known problems
● Breathing	Known chronic bronchitic Smokes "roll ups"; sister unable to say how many; thought to be "quite a number"
● Eating and drinking	Said to eat "fairly well" High alcohol intake : had been referred to psychiatrist but declined treatment
● Eliminating	No known problems
● Personal cleansing and dressing	"Scruffy" appearance Looks give the impression he did not look after himself very well
● Controlling body temperature	
● Mobilising	Usually active : no previous problems with mobility
● Working and playing	Unemployed : made redundant two years ago Public house predominates in social life
● Expressing sexuality	Close ties with mother, brother & sister Wife kept in contact since separation Has access to two children Hopes to die re-united with wife
● Sleeping	No known problems
● Dying	

Fig. 11.5   Patient Assessment Form: assessment of ALs (pre-admission status provided by family)

12
Conclusion

In this concluding chapter we discuss a number of issues and ideas which were suggested to us as a result of the studies presented by the contributors. In order to help readers follow this discussion, with its frequent reference back to the contributed chapters, a brief summary of each of the nine studies follows.

Summary of the nine studies

A study of a diabetic patient was undertaken by the sister of a diabetic unit, in conjunction with a nurse teacher who was conversant with the nursing process and the model for nursing. The study is of a 15-year-old boy, newly diagnosed as having diabetes mellitus. Nursing plans presented within the chapter consider both short-term goals for his nursing during the brief inpatient stay, and long-term goals for subsequent outpatient management. Data from two assessments carried out within the ward are presented as well as those from a third assessment undertaken two weeks after discharge to assess initial progress at home. An obvious focus of this study is the place of patient education in nursing. Among other things the authors comment in their discussion that the model for nursing, with its focus on activities of living, certainly aids identification of areas requiring planned teaching — an increasingly relevant type of nursing intervention.

A study in a surgical ward concerns the pre- and postoperative nursing over a ten-day period of hospitalisation of a 53-year-old woman admitted for cholecystectomy. The AL framework for assessment was found to be helpful, ensuring that the patient was viewed as a 'whole person'. Other nurses on the ward also liked the Patient Assessment Form as it provided more information than was usually available, for example mentioning the relevant fact that the patient had a handicapped son. A feature of the documentation included in this chapter is the use that was made of standard nursing plans. These, based on the AL framework, were used in conjunction with individual plans for the patient. The student nurse who carried out this study, with the guidance of a nursing lecturer, found that the mode of thinking encouraged by the model was a useful one. It promoted a wider view of nursing's contribution to a patient's care.

A health visitor's study of a mother and baby was able to consider only the initial few weeks of what is, in nursing terms, a lengthy contact between nurse and client. The health visitor who undertook this study was already employing the nursing process in her work and she describes this development in the first part of her chapter. She had considerable reservations initially about the relevance of the Roper, Logan and Tierney model for this aspect of her work. This was partly because the model seemed to focus on an individual (when her concern is with a baby, mother and family) and appeared to her to be oriented to the hospital setting (rather than community) and to patients during illness (as opposed to healthy people). However, adopting the AL framework for assessment was found to provide a very valuable approach. Because of this, part of the chapter is devoted to comment on each of the ALs in turn to focus on their relevance to a health visitor's work with mothers and children.

A midwife's study of a mother and baby was carried out by a student midwife under the supervision of a clinical teacher and in collaboration with a Director of Nurse Education. The study, in a postnatal ward, concerned a young woman who had given birth to her first child, a healthy baby girl. It was found that the AL framework for assessment encouraged a comprehensive assessment to be undertaken. It was felt that this contributed to the establishment of unusually good rapport between nurse and mother. In addition, some problems were identified which otherwise may have gone unnoted. Included in the documentation presented is a standard care plan based on the ALs which the authors suggest could be tried out and, once finalised, used by midwives in postnatal care.

A study of an elderly patient involved a 67-year-old woman, disabled by disseminated sclerosis. She had been admitted to the ward of a geriatric hospital for urinary investigations, continence training and rehabilitation. The two ward sisters who worked together on this study had already been using the process of nursing; examples of the proforma they employed are included in the chapter. However, they found the Patient Assessment Form, which reflects the thinking behind the model, an even more useful approach to nursing assessment. The form alerted them to identify the patient's abilities as well as disabilities, and to consider her previous life-style as well as her circumstances immediately prior to admission. There was some initial difficulty in designing a nursing plan using the AL framework; in the end a separate sheet was used for each AL. The result is shown in the documentation accompanying the chapter.

A study in a medical ward was carried out by the sister and one of the staff nurses. The nursing process had been introduced into the ward, and some of the problems experienced and the solutions found are discussed in the introduction to their chapter. The patient selected for the study employing the Roper, Logan and Tierney model was a 48-year-old man. He had myeloma; his condition deteriorated rapidly and, a month or so after admission to the ward, he died. A total of four assessments undertaken using the AL framework are detailed. These show a clearly identifiable change in this patient's condition over the period of the study. Following each assessment is a statement of problems, goals and plans. Although the authors found the model relatively easy in theory, they discuss the difficulties they had in documenting data according to ALs in a concise and logical manner.

A study in a psychiatric ward concerned a woman of 86 years of age. She was admitted to the psychiatric ward from sheltered housing for assessment of an organic brain syndrome because her condition had been giving rise to anxiety. The study spans a two-week period. In their presentation of the study, the authors (a staff nurse and nurse tutor) describe their initial apprehension about carrying out assessment using the AL framework. They had been accustomed to considering topics such as 'memory', 'orientation', 'thinking and perception'. However, they found the new approach did seem to be relevant for assessment of a psychiatric patient. It was even advantageous in directing attention to the patient's independence as well as dependence. The authors were sufficiently impressed with the potential of the model in psychiatric nursing to recommend further studies of its application.

A study of a patient at home was undertaken by a district nursing sister in collaboration with a lecturer in nursing studies who is also a qualified district nurse tutor. The patient was a 41-year-old woman who was suffering from cancer of the lung and requiring constant nursing. She had a husband and two teenage daughters. The care of this patient was shared by nurses and relatives and, in the chapter, it is described how the

family contributed to planning and recording the nursing required. Presentation of assessment data and nursing plans shows the complexity and diversity of this patient's problems and nursing needs. The documentation involved a consideration of all ALs and continuation sheets were used so that the minimum of additional writing was required at each assessment. The authors provide detailed comment on the Patient Assessment Form, pointing out some additional items of information which are required for use of the form in the community. Overall it was felt that the model for nursing did work in practice and is a relevant approach for community nursing. It was seen as helpful to the nursing officer when allocating staff, of great benefit to relief nurses, and a potentially effective tool for learners.

A study in a neurosurgical ward concerns a 38-year-old man who had suffered severe head injury after a fall. He was cared for in the intensive therapy unit for the first ten days. The study spans the ensuing two weeks spent in the ward before the patient's return to the referring hospital. The patient was still unconscious on admission to the ward. The admission assessment of ALs by the nurse was complemented by a profile of the patient drawn up on the basis of information about ALs obtained from relatives. The documentation included in the chapter shows how assessment, problems, goals and evaluation were recorded together on one form. The nursing plan was written down separately so that it could be kept at the patient's bedside and intervention was recorded on that form. The ward sister and senior nursing officer who collaborated on this study comment favourably on the model. However, they point out that the amount of time and effort necessary for its wider application in a ward should not be underestimated.

General comments on the nine studies

As we became increasingly familiar with the studies we realised the wealth of information which they have provided. There were several topics which we thought could be used for discussion, so as examples, we selected a few of them and below we give a short comment on each before discussing in more detail four other subjects.

Communication between nurses
In several of the studies it is evident that use of the Patient Assessment Form and nursing plans resulted in better communication between staff members, especially those on different shifts (surgical study, Ch. 4). Also in Chapter 4 it was reported that the patient's 30-year-old mentally handicapped son did not become an embarrassment to his mother because all the nurses knew about him and were interested in him. When he visited she was 'happy to see him accepted'. In comparison, this study commented on the 'lack of

communication' after looking at notes from a previous admission which merely informed members of staff that the patient had 'slept well'; had had a 'usual day' and had been 'up and about'. The elderly patient (Ch. 7) felt that all members of the nursing staff knew about her 'as a person'. The point is made in the district nursing study (Ch. 10) that new nurses did not have to ask the patient questions, but seemed 'to know about her'.

Considering the importance attached to the subject of 'communication' in nursing journals, the fact that practising nurses made the above comments about use of the Patient Assessment Form and nursing plans is especially encouraging.

Rapport between patients and staff

The midwifery study (Ch. 6) is the only one in which the actual word 'rapport' is used and it comments very favourably on this being established between the student midwife and the postnatal mother. But without exception all nine patients and their relatives were positive about the relationship which was established between themselves and members of the nursing staff who attributed this to the personalised approach encouraged by using the Patient Assessment Form.

Information about the family

The simple assessment form was designed to reflect the model for nursing. Although it has the word 'patient' in its title, it is encouraging that all contributors collected information about other members of the family when this was relevant. The district nursing study (Ch. 10) contains considerable information in the text and in the documentation, not only about the husband and two daughters but also about the patient's sister-in-law, and it similarly mentions the neighbours who visited frequently. The relevance of the knowledge that the husband was unemployed is shown in the midwifery study (Ch. 6). And all the staff in the neurosurgical ward were aware that the patient's 'sister and brother accepted the situation, but they shielded the mother from its gravity' (Fig. 11.2, p.161).

The health visitor (Ch. 5) took time to realise that not only information about the baby, but also information about the parents and siblings could be included on the Patient Assessment Form when collecting data about ALs (Fig. 5.1, p. 61).

Privacy for assessment

For the collection of assessment data it is stated in one contribution (Ch. 6) that a single room was considered desirable to provide the necessary privacy. But one of the studies (Ch. 8) was carried out in a Nightingale ward which could be said to afford less privacy than a single room. Consequently, in the multi-bedded areas, nurses will need to take precautions to afford the patient privacy, and for those patients/clients who have impaired hearing a single room can be reserved, even if it is an office.

Preventive aspects of nursing

Several of the studies stated that having to think about a patient's potential health problems when using the Patient Assessment Form acknowledged and emphasised the need for consideration of preventive nursing interventions. The surgical study (Ch. 4) not only recorded nursing interventions to prevent respiratory complications and deep venous thrombosis, but it also made the point that the mode of thinking encouraged by the concept of potential problems 'helped both the patient and her family to appreciate the need for self-care'. The diabetic boy was unaware of the precautions he should take regarding his feet (Fig. 3.2, p. 24) so an appointment was made for him to visit the chiropodist. And, of course where appropriate in several of the studies, the nursing interventions for prevention of pressure sores are recorded.

The model as a learning tool

By the nature of the project, those contributors who had no prior knowledge of the model could be said to have 'limited experience' of using it. Even so, in the surgical study (Ch. 4) the student nurse wrote: '. . . detailed nursing care plans . . . were good teaching aids for students and pupil nurses'. The student midwife (Ch. 6) considered that use of the model had been 'a real learning experience'; it had been 'rewarding' and 'stimulating' and had resulted in a 'sense of satisfaction'. The writers of the medical study (Ch. 8) after considering the extra documentation involved, wondered if use of the model can become a practical proposition, 'or will it be used merely as a learning exercise?' Yet later in their study they write '. . . it could be a useful tool for both teaching and using . . .' In the psychiatric study (Ch. 9) the contributors were 'sufficiently impressed with the potential of the model to suggest further studies'. The district nursing study (Ch. 10) records that the nursing officer considered the model 'a teaching tool' which could be used 'in the basic programme for registration and for student district nurses'. It is reassuring that the 'learning' referred to above took place in the clinical areas in which the studies were carried out.

Use of the word 'nursing'

The studies, in common with current nursing literature, use certain words and terms which have become associated with the process of nursing. In our books we avoided using the terms 'nursing care' and 'nursing care plans'. Our rationale for this is that in a shortened form, the word 'care' is more frequently used than the word 'nursing'. This is evidenced in some of the studies and in the nursing journals, and it takes determined effort not to omit the word 'nursing', but we are of the opinion that wherever possible the word 'nursing' should be used on its own.

Conceptual frameworks

Deliberately we did not use the concept of need in our model and explained why in some detail in Chapter 2 of *The Elements of Nursing*. We also stated that throughout the book the 'focus of living and nursing is not on needs but on the ALs because they are the behavioural manifestations of basic human needs'. The word 'need' occurs in several of the contributed studies but we did not change it. However, we would commend to readers that the use of any published conceptual framework for nursing demands interpretation of the framework/model as it is specified by the authors.

In spite of all the trials and trauma experienced by the contributors during the project and even until submission of the final manuscript, several of them state that they would be interested in further trials of the model!

Having reflected on the experience of the contributors and the content of the nine studies, we feel that readers should share some of our thoughts. Therefore to conclude this chapter we will discuss in more detail four subjects which seemed to us to merit further consideration:

- the activities of living as a framework for assessment
- goal setting and evaluation
- documentation
- our reflections on the model for nursing.

The activities of living as a framework for assessment

The model for nursing, as described in Chapter 2, is based on a model of living which has as its focus twelve *activities of living* (ALs). As a reminder these are: maintaining a safe environment; communicating; breathing; eating and drinking; eliminating; personal cleansing and dressing; controlling body temperature; mobilising; working and playing; expressing sexuality; sleeping; dying.

In applying the model, these activities of living are used as the framework for assessment of the patient by the nurse. The Patient Assessment Form (Fig 2.4, pp. 16-17) was designed to reflect this intention: the twelve ALs are listed on the right-hand side of the form for entering data from assessment.

The objectives in collecting data about a patient's ALs are to discover:

- previous routines
- what the patient can do for himself
- what the patient cannot do for himself
- problems (actual/potential) and previous coping mechanisms.

In trying out the model with the selected patient, the contributors were directed to carry out their nursing assessment using activities of living as the framework and to

document the data collected on the Patient Assessment Form. Contributors had been given a copy of *The Elements of Nursing* so that they could become familiar with the model for nursing and, specifically, the twelve activities of living. Guidelines for assessment of the ALs are included in the summary charts at the end of each AL chapter of the book (these are collected together in Appendix 1 of this book). We envisaged that these summary charts would be useful as an aide memoire to assessment and, in fact, contributors were given a photocopied set of the charts along with a photocopy of the first two chapters of *Learning to Use the Process of Nursing* in which guidance about assessment of ALs and use of the Patient Assessment Form are provided.

In the time available to prepare for their study we did not expect contributors to have become completely familiar with the AL framework for assessment. Indeed, the initial difficulties which they experienced in using this framework appear to have been due largely to uncertainty about exactly what information 'fitted in' to which AL heading on the form. These difficulties will be discussed later in this section.

But first, the reported advantages will be described. It seems appropriate to start with these because, without exception, contributors stated that they found the approach to be a relevant and advantageous one.

ADVANTAGES

One of the basic intentions of this book was to put to the test our belief that the model for nursing is applicable to all branches of nursing and all types of patients, irrespective of age and health/illness status. Although only a small number of studies are involved, they do span a variety of nursing settings and situations. It is an important outcome of the project that the AL framework for assessment did appear to provide a relevant and manageable approach for all of the patients who were involved. Indeed without exception the contributors identify advantages they discovered in the AL framework in comparison to their usual practice.

In the study of a diabetic patient (Ch. 3) it is mentioned that recording of assessment data in the AL framework produced a much more informative assessment than was formerly available. In their study in a surgical ward (Ch. 4) the comment is made that the AL approach was helpful in ensuring that the patient was looked at as a 'whole person'. The health visitor (Ch. 5) had initial reservations but discovered that the framework did encourage a comprehensive assessment of the baby involved in her study. Similarly, the report of the midwife's study of a mother and baby (Ch. 6) mentions that the AL approach helped to elicit information that might otherwise have been missed. For example, from assessing the AL of communicating, the mother's anxiety and apprehension about handling her new baby was identified.

In addition to encouraging a more comprehensive assessment, several contributors comment that the AL framework alerted them to discover the patient's abilities as well as disabilities. For example, the ward sisters who undertook the study of an elderly patient (Ch. 7) discovered how many personal cleansing and dressing activities the patient could manage in spite of her severe disablement from disseminated sclerosis. Those contributors also mention how useful it was to be directed to take account of the patient's previous lifestyle and not just her circumstances immediately prior to admission. The advantages of being reminded to look at the patient's independence are also acknowledged in the study of a patient in a psychiatric ward (Ch. 9): the contributors comment that the AL framework made them very aware of the need to preserve the patient's independence and, therefore, self-esteem.

The potential of the AL framework for assessment to focus on the *person* rather than the 'patient' is given recognition in a number of comments contained in the studies: 'I like the emphasis which this encourages, looking at the individual as a whole person rather than a collection of body systems' (Ch. 5: health visiting study); '. . . Many pieces of information about the patient were collected and these were certainly useful to know in order to . . . understand him more completely . . .. In general we find that the concept of ALs encourages a more thoughtful and thorough approach to the patient, seeing him as an individual with many needs and problems, not all necessarily directly related to his disease condition' (Ch. 8: medical nursing study).

Some contributors actually attribute the nurse's concern with the patient as an individual within this framework as at least partly responsible for increased patient satisfaction. The authors of the study in a surgical ward (Ch. 4) record the fact that the patient 'actually stated that she felt much more welcome than on her previous admission to hospital'. The midwifery study (Ch. 6) reports that the more detailed and person-oriented assessment procedure led to excellent communication between the mother and student midwife and the end result for the patient was a reduction in anxiety and a sense of satisfaction. The study of an elderly patient (Ch. 7) mentions how useful it was to have collected data about the AL of working and playing. This provided a talking point in conversation with the patient. The authors report that 'the patient felt all members of the nursing staff were interested in her as a person, not just as a patient'.

Some of the contributors describe reactions of their colleagues to the Patient Assessment Form. A detailed discussion of this aspect is included in the report of the study of a patient at home (Ch. 10). District nursing colleagues decided, after initial reservations, that 'use of the twelve ALs would really be beneficial when carrying out patient assessments . . . would provide a clearer picture of the patient, the family and the home situation'. Part-time district nurses were even more enthusiastic and saw the increased amount of information available to be of particular help to them. In this study, a relief nurse had taken over the patient's nursing for a few days and it is reported that this nurse 'felt she knew the

patient very well before she even met her because the assessments were so precise'. As the writers of that chapter point out, this must surely be beneficial to the patient as well as the nurse.

In that same chapter, the AL framework for assessment is commended for its potential as a teaching tool for students. Some of the studies had actually involved student nurses as participants. For example, in the midwifery study (Ch. 6), it was mentioned that the project had proved to be a valuable learning experience for the student midwife, 'producing a greater understanding of the various needs of both mother and baby'. The authors of the study in a neurosurgical ward (Ch. 11) actually asked some students undertaking the intensive care course in their hospital to use the Patient Assessment Form as part of an assignment. Despite considerable initial apprehension, the students found the framework to be a useful and helpful method of collecting information: 'All agreed that they had learned much more than usual about their patient and had therefore been better able to support and care for both the patient and the family.'

So, overall, the AL framework for assessment did prove to be a relevant and advantageous approach to the first stage in the process of nursing. This seemed to be true in all of the settings in which the model was tried out in this project. Certainly we had found that the framework worked well in the patient studies we prepared for *Learning to Use the Process of Nursing*, the sequel to our first book *The Elements of Nursing*. Indeed reviews of the second book have particularly commended its usefulness with respect to nursing assessment based on the AL framework.

We believe that it is absolutely essential for the process of nursing to be embodied in a conceptual model for nursing. We wholeheartedly endorse the statement made in the district nursing study (Ch. 10): 'The process of nursing is in itself merely a methodical and logical way of thinking. . . In itself it is inanimate; it is the use of a model for nursing that gives it purpose and meaning.'

INITIAL DIFFICULTIES

As mentioned in the introduction to this section about the AL framework for assessment, we did expect contributors to experience some difficulties initially because they had a relatively short time in which to become familiar with the details of the twelve ALs. And indeed in a number of studies, initial uncertainty about categorisation of data collected within the AL headings is recorded. Some found this more of a problem than others. The sister who carried out the study of a diabetic patient (Ch. 3), although initially concerned whether all necessary observations could be fitted into the twelve headings, found in practice that this turned out to be relatively easy to overcome by referring to guidelines in *The Elements of Nursing*.

The health visitor (Ch. 5) found it more difficult. She

describes how she was accustomed to categorising information by topics, such as 'feeding', 'immunisation', 'hygiene' and 'mother-baby relationship'. At first she felt it would be unworkable to change to the AL categorisation, mainly because she realised that some topics span more than one AL. The example of sterilising bottles is cited. Although obviously related to the AL of maintaining a safe environment, it is also closely linked to the AL of eating and drinking. Likewise, the information that the mother smoked could be mentioned under the ALs of maintaining a safe environment, and breathing.

In the study of a psychiatric patient (Ch. 9), the authors describe similar difficulties in transferring to the AL framework from their accustomed method of recording information about a patient. They wondered about where to 'fit in' under AL headings information about such things as 'memory', 'orientation', 'thinking and perception'. But they appreciated that these are cerebral functions and are therefore associated with the AL of communicating. It is perhaps pertinent to mention that we appreciate the considerable amount of data which may be relevant to this AL in some nursing contexts, psychiatric nursing being one. There was concern, too, about where to record findings of psychiatric disorder such as delusions, disorientation and hallucinations. However, once they accepted that such findings would not fit naturally under one heading, but would appear under several headings in different contexts, such problems became easier to deal with. For example, notes of the patient's disorientation in time and place were relevant under both the AL of maintaining a safe environment ('she could wander off and become lost') and communicating ('she was occasionally unaware of her surroundings and the nurses' identity').

Initially the district nurses (Ch. 10) thought that it would be necessary to supplement the twelve AL headings with some others if all necessary information was to be recorded. For example, an additional heading of 'economic factors' was considered until it was realised that relevant details of the patient's financial circumstances could be put within the AL of working and playing on the rationale that income is usually related to work. Details of facilities in the home are very important to record in district nursing. However, instead of adding a separate section, it was decided that such details could be entered under several AL headings: toilet facilities under 'eliminating'; bathing facilities under 'personal cleansing and dressing'; cooking facilities under 'eating and drinking'; and heating arrangements in the home under 'controlling body temperature'.

Realisation by the authors of this particular study, that a variety of factors do 'fit in' to the AL framework, is interesting. In developing our approach to assessment from the starting point of the model for nursing, we deliberately avoided fragmenting information about the patient by leaving out of the Form categories such as 'physical', 'psychological', 'social' and 'economic' factors and 'religious beliefs'. Because in reality such factors are inextricably linked with activities of living, we believed that they should be subsumed under each AL heading. The evidence that contributors came to realise that this could be done, and that it seems a reasonable and useful approach, lends support to our original thinking.

On the whole contributors to this book have reacted favourably to our list of twelve ALs. In developing the model of living we gave considerable thought to the number and description of items in the list of activities of living. We realised that most people could compose a list of everyday living activities and without doubt there would be common items in the lists such as breathing, eating and drinking, and mobilising. However we added several to the more commonly mentioned activities of living, for instance 'maintaining a safe environment', 'working and playing', 'expressing sexuality' and 'dying'.

The authors of the study of an elderly patient (Ch. 7) mention that it took them some time to think of 'maintaining a safe environment' as carrying out activities to prevent pollution, fire, accidents and infection. Yet they realised after reading the relevant chapter in *The Elements of Nursing* that all facets of this AL are indeed relevant to a geriatric unit. Also they had previously thought of 'controlling body temperature' as a purely physiological function and not as an activity of living. Then they appreciated that everyone, especially the elderly, must carry out activities (such as dressing appropriately and ensuring adequte heating) to assist this function. The AL of 'expressing sexuality' was another one which took some time for these contributors to appreciate as relevant but it made more sense to them when they began to consider ways in which masculinity and femininity are expressed.

The AL of expressing sexuality is probably the one in our list which has most often been commented on as a strange inclusion! The authors of the study in a neurosurgical ward (Ch. 11) allude to this. The intensive care course students who were given the Patient Assessment Form to try out, felt threatened by the questions that they imagined would be required to elicit the necessary information about some of the less familiar ALs, including 'expressing sexuality'. However, it turned out that their worries were unfounded. Perhaps it is the name of this AL that causes the initial difficulty. We did indeed have tremendous problems (and amusement) in deciding upon its title. But the important question is whether doubts about its inclusion in the AL list are dispelled once the relevant chapter in *The Elements of Nursing* (Ch. 16) has been studied. Nevertheless, it does need to be mentioned that minimal use has been made of the AL in the studies presented in this book. However, no strong case has been put to us so far that would cause us to go back on our initial decision to include 'expressing sexuality' in our list of ALs.

'Dying' is another AL which sometimes causes uncertainty. Strictly speaking it is not an activity, but an act. However, it is the final act of living and one which affects all other ALs. The rationale for including it in our list derives from the knowledge that comprehensive assessment of a dying patient and his relatives is an extremely important nursing activity. It was interesting to note that some of the contributors saw the relevance of including 'dying' in the AL list even although the patient was unlikely to die. In the health visiting study (Ch. 5) mention is made of situations in which the subject might be raised: for example, if there has been a previous stillbirth or infant death, or if there is anxiety about the possibility of a cot death. The authors of the study of an elderly patient (Ch. 7) similarly mention that, although there was no relevant information to record for the AL of dying, its inclusion on the assessment form alerted them to the possibility that, had the patient wished it, she could have been encouraged to express her thoughts.

UNRESOLVED DIFFICULTIES

Difficulties with the AL framework for assessment which have been described so far mainly arose because of unfamiliarity with the model and the precise nature of the twelve activities of living. We appreciate that there was limited time available for the contributors to develop a complete understanding of the model. And, when using a model, one has to be conversant with it before applying it with confidence in practice. The interrelatedness of activities of living does result in initial uncertainty about the categorisation of specific types of patient data under AL headings. In addition, there is the need to recognise which body structure and function we had associated with each AL. However, even assuming that contributors had appreciated all the complexities of the model, some real difficulties could have emerged in the course of trying out the model in the 'real world'. As it was, only three topics appear to have been a problem in the recording of data from assessment of activities of living under the twelve AL headings. These were *pain, haemorrhage* and *pressure sores*.

Difficulty in dealing with the first two of these was raised in the study in a surgical ward (Ch. 4). Where should 'pain' be considered and recorded when using the AL framework for assessment? Pain can affect functioning in all ALs, but it was felt that assessment of pain ought also to be considered in terms of how the patient felt about the pain. The authors quote Hunt (1979): 'Pain is what the patient says that it is.' So does that suggest assessment of pain essentially comes under assessment of the AL of 'communicating'?

Difficulties with categorising pain were also experienced in the study of a patient at home (Ch. 10). The contributors question whether pain should be assessed in relation to various activities of living. However, several examples of pain not directly associated with any one AL are given: headache, angina at rest and abdominal pain not related to elimination. By referring back to *The Elements of Nursing* the contributors realised that pain could be categorised appropriately within the AL of 'communicating', but that initially this possibility had not seemed obvious to them. Perhaps it would, had it been remembered that the nervous system is part of the body structure and function related to the AL of communicating in *The Elements of Nursing*.

However, we chose to write about pain in that book as a separate entity within the chapter on 'Biological aspects of living' (Ch. 3). The rationale for this was that pain can affect any of the activities of living and a general understanding of the physiology and perception of pain, reaction to and assessment of pain, is essential for all nurses. We then identified and discussed particular types of pain in relation to the ALs individually in the latter part of the book, including this in the section which was called 'Discomforts associated with the AL of . . .'

The difficulties noted by the contributors have certainly alerted us to the possibility that clearer guidance about the assessment of pain, and documentation of related information within the ALs, may be necessary. This is something we will reconsider when preparing a new edition of *The Elements of Nursing*. In general, we would suggest that pain specifically relating to a particular AL should be considered and documented as such on the Patient Assessment Form. Pain not specifically related to any one AL, and the patient's perception of pain, could be linked to the AL of 'communicating' for purposes of assessment and problem identification.

Similar difficulty over *haemorrhage* was raised by the authors of the study in a surgical ward. They considered that haemorrhage (internal and external) had no obvious association with any one AL and so were unable to categorise related information within the AL framework.

Interestingly 'haemorrhage' does not appear as such in the index to *The Elements of Nursing*. Admittedly it is included as a cause of shock, and the phenomenon of shock is described as one of the body defence mechanisms in Chapter 3, 'Biological aspects of living'. There is too, a reference to postoperative wound observation — to check for bleeding — in Chapter 12 about the AL of personal cleansing and dressing. In addition a specific type of haemorrhage — haemoptysis — is mentioned in Chapter 9 dealing with the AL of breathing and there is another brief mention of haemorrhage related to respiration rate.

Because we were using an activities of living framework rather than a 'body systems' approach, relevant anatomy and physiology is presented in *The Elements of Nursing* as 'The body structure and function required for the AL of . . .'. In the AL of breathing, this section deals with the respiratory system (pulmonary aspects of the cardiopulmonary system) and the circulatory system (cardiovascular aspects of the cardiopulmonary system). Logically having placed the circulatory system within the AL of breathing, haemorrhage should have been discussed in more detail in that chapter (Ch. 9) instead of in Chapter 3.

This observation about haemorrhage by the contributors of the surgical nursing study is an important one. The nurse was alerted to haemorrhage as a potential problem for the patient because it is included on the standard postoperative plan they devised (Fig. 4.4, pp. 42-43). But the question is raised as to whether, without this, the nurse might have neglected to carry out related assessment and to identify haemorrhage as a potential problem. We are grateful to have had this difficulty brought to our attention and clearly we must give careful consideration to it when preparing a new edition of *The Elements of Nursing*.

The third topic which appeared to present unresolved difficulties in the context of the AL framework was *pressure sores*. In the study of a patient at home (Ch. 10) it is pointed out that relevant ALs included 'eliminating', 'personal cleansing and dressing' and 'eating and drinking'. Yet, because of the association between pressure sores and immobility, the authors of this study decided to assess pressure sores under the AL of 'mobilising'.

Care of pressure areas was an important aspect of the nursing of the patient in the study in a medical ward (Ch. 8). The two authors found themselves in disagreement about where in the AL framework the assessment of the problem of pressure sores should be placed. Would they record relevant information under 'maintaining a safe environment' or 'mobilising' or 'eating and drinking' or 'eliminating'? They comment however that the choice of heading was not their main concern. What did worry them was the possibility that such important information as pressure area status could be missed altogether because the relevant data may be dispersed among several ALs.

In *The Elements of Nursing* our discussion of pressure sores was placed in the chapter about the AL of personal cleansing and dressing (Ch. 12) because the skin was seen as the body structure relevant to this AL and pressure sores are one form of loss of skin continuity. In the summary chart at the end of the chapter 'degree of risk of pressure sores' is included in the list of topics for assessment and 'pressure sores' noted within the list of patients' problems. However, the data from assessment which can lead to identification of pressure sores as a potential problem do derive from a variety of other ALs, as pointed out by contributors. This example serves to emphasise the interrelatedness of activities of living. The difficulty seems to be not one of assessment, but of stating pressure sores as a potential problem within the AL framework. It seems to us logical for this problem to be categorised within the AL of personal cleansing and dressing. However, we appreciate that related data may be contained elsewhere in the assessment form. Attention could be drawn to this in the nursing plan because inevitably the goals set, the intervention planned and the evaluation will all take account of the various ALs concerned.

CHECKLIST FOR ASSESSMENT OF ALs

The right-hand side of the Patient Assessment Form, for assessment of ALs, only contains the AL headings. The assumption is that to be fully conversant with all twelve ALs and the relevant body structure and function is a necessary

prerequisite to carrying out assessment using the AL framework. This necessitates study of *The Elements of Nursing* and reference can be made as an aide memoire to the summary charts at the end of the AL chapters.

However, the reports of the nine studies in this book remind us that to become familiar with our AL framework does take time. We have appreciated that it is perhaps more difficult to become familiar with this framework when a different approach has previously been employed. Some of the initial difficulties which contributors found, clearly arose from the fact that they were used to assessing and documenting within categories different from ALs. Therefore it is not surprising that nurse learners, unfamiliar with using any one particular approach, seemed to have found less difficulty with the framework.

In the study in a surgical ward (Ch. 4) the authors point out that the semi-structured approach to assessment implicit in the nature of the AL framework does give scope to the prepared and perceptive interviewer. However, comparing the Patient Assessment Form with structured proforma, they note that because the form contains no sub-headings or specific questions, it is impossible to know whether questions were asked or observations made in a particular area.

In the report of the district nursing study (Ch. 10), mention is made of the decision taken to devise a checklist for assessment. The result is shown in Figure 10.2 (p. 139). It consists of a series of 'triggers' to the memory in relation to each AL.

Having reflected on this example, and considered the difficulties encountered in using the AL framework for assessment, we wondered if a checklist for each AL might be useful as an adjunct to the Patient Assessment Form. However we consider there are disadvantages in that the nurse may become committed to the narrowness of the specific content of the list, rather than the broad underlying principles. We would prefer that nurses develop an approach to assessment based on *The Elements of Nursing* and *Learning to Use the Process of Nursing*.

IDENTIFICATION OF PROBLEMS

The end point of assessment of ALs is identification of problems. The extreme right-hand side of the Patient Assessment Form has a column for identified problems to be listed. Differentiation of 'actual' problems and 'potential' problems is intended.

Very few difficulties were experienced by contributors in the task of problem identification and statement of problems on the Patient Assessment Form. Examination of all of the completed forms shows that it is possible to state problems concisely, yet unambiguously, and to accomplish this within the AL framework of the model. The authors of the study of an elderly patient (Ch. 7) comment how useful they found it to be able to see at a glance the patient's problems.

Contributors appear to have grasped without difficulty the distinction between actual and potential problems. The health visitor (Ch. 5) comments on her initial uncertainty about how many of the possible potential problems, relevant in the context of her preventive role and the long-term nature of her involvement, should be listed on the Patient Assessment Form. Her decision to include only those specifically suggested by data from assessment of that baby seems an appropriate one (Fig. 5.1, p. 61).

That contributor also discussed the need to recognise any difference in perception of problems between nurse and client. In *Learning to Use the Process of Nursing* we used the terms 'patient-perceived problem' and 'nurse-perceived problem' to describe this difference. It is an important consideration because, as mentioned in the section on 'Evaluation' below, it affects what goals are set, and that requires close collaboration between nurse and patient if intervention is to be effective.

The process of nursing is essentially a 'problem-solving approach'. We have incorporated this idea into the model by focusing on *problems* related to activities of living. The use of the word 'problems', however, does risk attracting the criticism that our model is concerned more with 'cure' than prevention of ill-health and promotion of health. In describing the model in *The Elements of Nursing* the case was made for considering 'problems' rather than 'needs'. We emphasised that we view nursing as helping patients to *solve, alleviate, cope with* or *prevent* problems related to activities of living. The studies presented in this book have reassured us that concern with a patient's 'problems' does not preclude consideration of goals related to prevention of ill-health and promotion of health. More is said about this in the following discussion.

Goal setting and evaluation

The phases of the process in the model for nursing are so interrelated that only for purposes of description can they be separated. As an example of the interrelatedness, evaluation could be said to start whenever a goal is stated for each identified problem, actual or potential. The written goal (set on the basis of assessment data) is the criterion which will be used later to evaluate whether or not the intervention has been effective. Goal setting then, is an integral part of evaluation; without written goals, evaluation is a misnomer.

Evaluation is often viewed as the most difficult part of the process. Appreciation of the fact that evaluation is essentially linked with written goals 'stated wherever possible in observable and/or measurable terms' (*The Elements of Nursing*, p. 67) may help nurses to develop the necessary skills for evaluating. Indeed in the diabetic study (Fig. 3.3, p. 26) having the column for recording goals alongside that for evaluation shows clearly that these contributors realised the

interrelatedness of the two phases of the process of nursing. And in the surgical study (Fig. 4.3, pp. 40-41) the column which has the heading 'Goal and goal criteria' shows very well that those who compiled the preoperative nursing plans were aware of the essential fact that goal setting provides the criteria for evaluation.

It is important that there is discussion 'with the patient whenever possible, and perhaps with his family and neighbours about the feasible goals which can be anticipated' (*The Elements of Nursing*, p. 67). Evidence in the studies that this part of the model was used has reassured us that application of the process part of the model does not result in goals being imposed on patients. Even for an unconscious patient in a neurosurgical ward (Ch. 11) mention is made of the involvement of the contributors with the patient's family before goal setting. For instance, before writing the goal at the AL of communicating, 'to anticipate needs by careful observation' the contributors knew that there had previously been 'no known problems' with this AL (Fig. 11.5, p. 164). The phrase 'patient's own goal' appears on the individual nursing plan (Fig. 4.5, p. 44) in relation to gradual weight reduction, and this provides further reassurance that the contributors had no difficulty in interpreting this important part of the model.

In the columns headed goals (diabetic study, Fig. 3.3, p. 26) there are examples of goals being stated in a health promotion context. For example, 'feels happy and relaxed in the ward' and 'feels fit and well' are written in the column for short-term goals and we would emphasise that they did not arise from a problem per se. And there are examples in the column for long-term goals, 'accepts diabetes as an inconvenience which he controls while leading a normal life' and 'performs work of his choice confidently and takes any exercise he likes'. To achieve these broadly stated goals, it is obvious from the study that the intervention planned was education; and the contributors comment favourably on use of the model to discover which areas of living require 'health education'. They wrote: 'Since nurses have a responsibility for health education, the model for nursing certainly permits the detection of those areas requiring planned help.' In the health visiting study (Fig. 5.5, p. 67) there is an example of the health promoting goal of a 'contented baby' being set to solve the actual problem of 'over stimulation' of the baby. Another example relates to the mother; the health promoting goal of 'decreased anxiety' was set to alleviate, solve or help the mother cope with the actual problem of 'maternal anxiety'.

The health visiting study (Fig. 5.5, p. 67) also gives examples of two goals which are preventive in nature; to deal with the actual problem of 'immunisation default' the goal of 'completed schedule' was set. Every living person has a potential problem of developing an infectious disease, but for some of the diseases immunisation is available to prevent/decrease the likelihood of the potential problem becoming an actual one. The other goal which is preventive in nature is 'no infection' related to the baby's potential problem of 'infection' developing in her engorged breasts. The preventive aspects of nursing ill patients resulting from identification of their potential as well as their actual problems, is well illustrated in the surgical study (Fig. 4.3, p. 41) as 'Potential complications related to surgery and anaesthesia'. This leads to goal setting and the statement of goal criteria to be used at evaluation. In contrast the midwifery study (Fig. 6.1, p. 73) identifies 'lack of bonding' as a potential problem and later records the outcome/evaluation as 'mother now confident and relaxed when looking after her baby'. It therefore seems reasonable for us to conclude that use of our model for nursing results in setting goals aimed at the promotion of health and the prevention of ill health, as well as the more generally understood aim of resolving actual health problems.

It has to be noted too that there can be differences between the nurse's and the patient's perception of a problem, which can affect goal setting and subsequent evaluation. There is an example in the health visiting study (Ch. 5) of the possible difference in perception between the health visitor and a mother, regarding the cause of her baby's nappy rash. The mother thinks that teething has caused the rash and the health visitor's assessment is that inadequate hygiene is the real cause. Skilful resolution of the perceptual difference, without creating resentment in the mother, is necessary so that she will see the need to implement the plan to achieve the goal with which she agrees, 'baby will have an intact healthy skin'. It was evident in the medical ward study (Ch. 8) that there was difference in perception about the gravity of the patient's illness between the patient and the contributors. They identified as a potential problem 'non-acceptance of diagnosis' for which their stated goal was 'encourage patient to talk about his health and become more accepting of actual/potential, short-/long-term implications'. The wording of that goal makes it a nursing intervention to achieve the goal, but re-wording would give a patient-descriptive goal, for example 'Patient more accepting of actual/potential, short-/long-term implications'. Wherever possible goals should be stated in terms of what the patient will achieve.

The health visiting study (Ch. 5) gives an instance when a problem did not lead to goal setting with subsequent evaluation, but resulted in recording 'no action taken'. This situation can arise when parents who complain about a child's poor sleeping pattern have taken the child into bed with them every night. The health visitor may find that such parents have no intention or inclination to 'do' anything themselves to establish a satisfactory sleeping pattern. 'All my advice and plans for the child are rendered nil because the parents are not prepared to implement them.' It may be unrealistic to set goals in such circumstances, but it is important to record the discussion.

This study gives an example of the complexity of goal setting and evaluation. It concerns two sets of parents; one had acted on the advice of the health visitor and had procured and used a fireguard; the other had not, but the outcome was that there had not been an accident in either home. In one instance a goal was achieved without acceptance of the proposed intervention; but in the other instance did the carrying out of the intervention procure the goal?

The discussion in this section, supported by relevant quotes from the studies illustrates how the contributors tackled goal setting and evaluation, thereby contributing substantially to knowledge about these two complex phases of the process of nursing implicit in the model.

Documentation

The objective when using nursing documents is that any nurse after reading them will have sufficient information about the patient to enable her to relate to him as a person and be conversant with the needed nursing interventions. With the inevitable changes in nursing staff this is a very important objective. Equally the new nurse needs to know the patient's previous routines of daily living so that she does not interfere unnecessarily with them. She needs to be aware of any health problems related to his ALs which means that she must know what he can and cannot do for himself; and she needs to know the planned nursing interventions to achieve the set goals. She must then be able to document additional assessment data, and record interventions and evaluations which she has carried out during her spell of duty. There is no argument against all this being an essential part of nursing, since no one nurse can be on duty throughout the 24 hours of each day, and sufficient detail about the patient cannot possibly be conveyed in verbal reports.

PATIENT ASSESSMENT FORM

All the contributors were asked to use the Patient Assessment Form which is illustrated and discussed in Chapter 2 of this book. All nine studies therefore contain an illustration of a completed Patient Assessment Form for the patient selected for the study. Most contributors considered that there was limited space for recording data and those with large handwriting are clearly at a disadvantage. It was suggested that a combination of these factors could lead to relevant information being omitted or to cramped and illegible handwriting. In revising the Form (Fig. 12.1, pp. 181-182) we have omitted the horizontal lines on the second page (p. 182) and used the AL headings as a checklist to overcome these difficulties.

Several of the contributors mentioned that familiarity with both the model and the Patient Assessment Form would help to solve the difficulties which they experienced about what goes where on each side of the form. And it has to be remembered that two essential nursing skills are writing only relevant information and doing so concisely. Throughout the nine studies there are more positive than negative comments about the form and there are several helpful suggestions for its modification.

Biographical and health data

The left-hand side of the original Patient Assessment Form is designed for collection of biographical and health data. In Chapter 2 of *Learning to Use the Process of Nursing* (which contributors had received before embarking on the project) some guidance was given about completion of this part of the form. It collects information about the home background which was found to be useful in several of the studies. In the surgical ward (Ch. 4) the information was used in planning the patient's discharge and it was also used indirectly to plan patient teaching in that it prompted the nurse to think of discharge goals.

A suggestion in the study of an elderly patient (Ch. 7) was that the contributors would have liked a space for a brief description of the patient to alert a new nurse as to what to expect on her first approach to the patient. Although the example given was factual, we see an inherent danger in that it could lead to 'labelling' which could be to the patient's disadvantage. At one stage in the project, the district nurses throught that a brief description would be helpful but they later discarded the idea on the grounds that the relief nurse was adequately pre-informed from reading the Patient Assessment Form (Ch. 10).

The district nurses suggested two extra items at 'type of accommodation' namely 'entry to accommodation' and 'deficiencies'. However, they know that they need this information and they agreed that the one prompt 'type of accommodation' could elicit the three different pieces of information which they require, but we will give guidance about this in the text of the next edition of *The Elements of Nursing*.

We gave careful consideration to a suggestion that an extra heading (prompt) was needed at which 'support services' could be recorded and we have done this. Such information may be needed for planning discharge and is almost always required by nurses in the community.

Another suggestion was to add 'family's perception of patient's health status' and this is needed; the extra prompt to elicit this useful information has been placed below 'patient's perception of current health status'.

In the midwifery study (Ch. 6) the contributors suggest that an extra section was needed in their specialty for recording prenatal care, length of labour, type of delivery and condition of baby at birth; they felt that it was inappropriate to record such information at the AL of expressing sexuality. But could these facts have been recorded at 'past medical history'?

During collection of data for the psychiatric study (Ch. 9) the contributors were of the opinion that they needed more space at 'past medical history' but realised that several of the patient's medical diagnoses were in fact duplicated, so with attention to this and handwriting, the space was adequate. The district nurses also foresaw possible difficulties at this section as many of their patients do have a long 'past medical history'.

Yet another suggestion was for the addition of 'appointments', 'transport' and 'equipment on loan'; these

would probably be useful on all forms and it could help to focus the nurse's attention to planning for the patient's/client's discharge from the health care system. This type of information could be recorded under 'Other Notes'.

Assessment of activities of living

The right-hand side of the original Patient Assessment Form relates directly to the model for nursing. The editors have been thinking about the model for at least five years and have become increasingly skilled at allocating information to particular ALs. However, working with the contributors and discussing with them the AL framework of the model, helping them to resist the idea that they needed a space for recording the patient's psychological status and his social status, reminded us of our early thinking about the model. It is only fair to remind readers that the project was carried out over a four month period and that only a few of the contributors had any prior knowledge of the model. Some of the initial difficulties which the experienced in documenting AL data have already been discussed in a previous section of this chapter.

In the surgical study (Ch. 4), the perceptive student nurse pointed out that she did not follow the order of the ALs on the form when carrying out the assessment. We had encouraged this in *Learning to Use the Process of Nursing* (p. 2) and it was reassuring that the student's interpretation of the model did not cause her to stick to a rigid formula, a criticism which some nurses make about the use of proforma for collection of data from patients.

The contributors of the study of a diabetic patient (Ch. 3) found it necessary to use the AL part of the assessment form on more than one occasion. Although it was relevant to include only six ALs on the nursing plan, they felt that all ALs needed to be assessed at intervals and these are referred to in the text as first assessment, second assessment and so on; the date at the top of the form alerts the nurse to the most recent assessment. In the medical study (Ch. 8) all ALs were assessed on four occasions, but there is discussion of the fact that, for instance, the data for maintaining a safe environment did not change, so there was repetitive writing leading to a bulky document. In the psychiatric ward (Ch. 9) three assessments of all ALs were carried out but it was found that the biographical and health data did not change so the biographical and health side of the form was thought of as a separate document. These then, are some of the ways in which contributors dealt with documentation of AL data.

Not all of the contributors bore in mind the objectives in collecting assessment data which are to discover the patient's/client's usual routines and what he can and cannot do in relation to his ALs. In two studies which did document this information at relevant ALs (elderly patient, Ch. 6; psychiatric ward, Ch. 9) comment was made on the usefulness of the information about what the patient could do independently, and that it helped the patient to retain her dignity and self-esteem.

The final point about assessment of ALs is identification of any problems which the patient has in relation to his ALs. The contributors did not seem to have great difficulty in finally deciding about the patient's problems, both actual and potential, related to his ALs, and this information is documented on the far right of the original Patient Assessment Form.

NURSING PLANS AND THEIR DOCUMENTATION

Documenting nursing plans and their implementation is undoubtedly the greatest challenge in the application of the model to practice. The nursing plan should not only inform the new nurse of the particular nursing interventions which have to be implemented during the spell of duty, but it should contain all the nursing interventions, for example, some interventions may only be carried out weekly but could have nursing implications in the intervening period; whereas the Patient Assessment Form tells her about the patient's previous routines, what he can and cannot do in relation to each AL. Both these documents are necessary as they complement each other.

Contributors had freedom of choice in designing their documents to record the planning, implementation and evaluation phases of the process. In their nursing plans, the majority of the contributors stated the goals for each actual and potential problem on the left side and put the column for evaluation on the right side, these being separated by the nursing intervention. On the surgical ward (Ch. 4) it was found necessary to have a separate page of nursing plan related to each problem. In the study of an elderly patient (Ch. 7) the problem, of unequal amounts of writing about implementation and evaluation for the problems associated with each AL, was solved by having a separate sheet for each AL. This solution also avoided repetitious writing of the AL headings, and separation of information about each AL. Avoidance of repetitious writing of AL headings in the nursing plans was also accomplished in the district nursing study (Figs 10.3.1, 2 and 3, pp. 140-145) and in the study of the diabetic patient (Fig. 3.2, pp. 24-25).

In an attempt to minimise documentation a standard care plan for use with postnatal mothers was developed (Fig. 6.5, p. 78), then only additional information would be written on an individual care plan. A similar suggestion is made in the study carried out in a diabetic unit (Ch. 3). And the contributors of the surgical study designed standard pre- and postoperative plans (Figs 4.3 and 4.4, pp. 40-43) which were used for the patient in the project, together with an individual nursing plan (Fig. 4.5, pp. 44-45). This idea could be developed further bearing in mind that they will need to be reliable, which can only be achieved by adequate trial, feedback and modification if necessary. A few standard plans have been published and we would encourage publication so that there can be ensuing discussion by nurses in nursing journals.

So far we have discussed two documents, the Patient Assessment Form and the Nursing Plan, each of which should give sufficient information to a new nurse to carry out the planned nursing interventions for each patient. But then assessment is not a once-only activity or a rigid routine carried out at a particular time; it is a continuous or ongoing activity and one of the difficulties experienced by the contributors was in deciding where the extra assessment data should be documented. Nor is the nursing plan a static thing but may require revision as additional data are collected from ongoing assessment, and evaluation reveals whether or not goals are being reached. The amount and frequency of documentation from assessment and evaluation will vary according to the type of patient. It will be frequent for example in the postoperative period, and may be less frequent for long-stay patients.

The carrying out of the planned nursing interventions has to be recorded on a third document, whatever it is called. For example if the nursing plan states 'two hourly turning' then the times at which the patient was turned on each shift are recorded on this third document. These jottings would be a 'daily report' on the patient; they are the notes of what happens to the patient during each shift. They are however essential data and should not be destroyed. We think that the term 'implementation sheet' is too constraining; also many nursing 'activities' are carried out which are not implementations of the planned nursing 'interventions'. Is this day-to-day flow chart the place to record the extra data as they are gathered by ongoing assessment? And if they reveal a problem, is the problem then recorded on the nursing plan with the date, followed by a goal, and the appropriate nursing intervention to achieve the goal? And is this day-to-day chart the place on which to record evaluation? If the goal has been achieved, is this then entered on the nursing plan with the date and cancellation of the nursing intervention? If the goal is not being achieved, are extra assessment data collected on this day-to-day chart, and if they suggest a change in nursing intervention, is this entered with the date on the nursing plan to achieve the original set goal? There will be occasions of goal non-achievement when, in the absence of extra assessment data, professional judgement is the base on which the nursing intervention is changed, although the original set goal is unchanged.

The contributors of the surgical study did develop a 'Progress/evaluation record' on which the day-to-day information is recorded under selected AL headings. We wonder if there is any benefit in using these headings; it certainly increase the writing (Fig. 4.7, p. 47). In our book *The Elements of Nursing* we wrote: 'A day-to-day record must be made of the nursing activities, when they were carried out, and by whom, together with any relevant information; for example, the patient may have experienced nausea while his wound dressing was being changed' (p. 68). At that time we did not envisage the day-to-day record being in AL format. In the other studies day-to-day information was recorded on the nursing plan and where the patient's stay was short as in the postnatal study, this did not result in undue writing (Fig. 6.3,

p. 75). In contrast it produced a very bulky, time-consuming document in the medical study (Ch. 8). Perhaps we will need to give more guidance about documentation of the planned nursing interventions — the implementation and evaluation phases of the process of nursing — in the next edition of *The Elements of Nursing*.

The Patient Assessment Form was designed to permit identification of the patient's/client's problems with their ALs, and the nurse responds to those which are amenable to nursing help. So the model and the form are about nursing: but there is a 'dependent component of nursing' described in *The Elements of Nursing* (p. 63) and examples are given of drugs, treatments and tests which are prescribed by the doctor to be carried out by the nurse. The documents we have discussed so far do not cater for the nursing interventions which derive from medical prescription and this presented a real difficulty to the contributors. But most hospitals and local authorities have a method of documenting prescribed drugs, the route by which they are given and the time of administration: and many hospitals use a TPR and BP chart. Nurses are well versed in the use of these two documents which they share with the medical staff. However these do not cater for other nursing interventions which derive from medical or other prescription and we now advocate a section for this purpose (p. 184).

Having shared our thoughts and those of the contributors with the readers we feel that no one will doubt the complexities of documenting nursing. Furthermore, it is time-consuming and involves much paper work. The search is therefore for simple documents which will adequately record the complex activity of nursing. The documents designed by the contributors and displayed throughout this book contain potential for refinement and adaptation and some of their suggestions have been incorporated in Figure 12.1. This is a modified edition of the original Patient Assessment Form which appeared in *The Elements of Nursing* and was used by the contributors to this book. The new form has only minor changes in the format for collection of biographical and health data, but the layout for documenting data collected from the assessment of the ALs has been changed. Instead of an allocated space for each AL with its name, as in the original form, most of the page is left blank to encourage the nurse to use the space to best advantage for that particular patient. There is however a list of the twelve ALs to act as a reminder of the scope of the assessment. We have also added a Nursing Plan which makes provision for documentation related to goals; nursing interventions related to ALs which identify the nurse-initiated contribution to health care; and evaluation. Finally there is a page for recording those nursing interventions derived from medical and other prescription.

Our original Patient Assessment Form permitted documentation of the assessment stage of the process of nursing ending with problem identification. The new format goes beyond that to the stage of evaluation of both nurse-initiated interventions and those derived from medical and other prescription.

Our reflections on the model for nursing

Since we originally presented the model for nursing based on a model of living in *The Elements of Nursing* we have continued to think about nursing within the conceptual framework of the models. As a result of this, together with the insight gained by our reflection on the studies presented in this book, we now think that minor modification of the models is appropriate. Readers are referred to Chapter 2 of this book in which both models are outlined.

THE ACTIVITIES OF LIVING

The models' focus on twelve activities of living is obviously relevant in nursing as testified by the contributors. It was reassuring to find that they were as useful in the studies of 'well' people (health visiting study, Ch. 5; midwifery study, Ch. 6), as in the studies of acutely ill patients, and in those carried out in long-term settings. We believe that this was due to the use in all the studies of the Patient Assessment Form which blends the model with the first phase of the process of nursing; it directs users to discover patients'/clients' usual routines, and what they can and cannot do independently in relation to their ALs.

Two of the studies paid tribute to this direction — in the psychiatric ward it was reported that since independence is a part of self-esteem and dignity it was important for the nurses to discover what the patient could still do. In the study of an elderly patient (Ch. 7) the contributors say that by being directed to find out what the patient could do, they were surprised at how many personal hygiene activities she could manage to carry out in spite of severe disability.

The assessment data about the twelve ALs are inspected with the objective of identifying where relevant, the patient's/client's actual and potential problems with any of the ALs. It is the inclusion of the concept of potential problems which permits the model/Patient Assessment Form to be applicable to 'well' people, in addition to 'ill' or 'handicapped' people, whether the illness or handicap is predominantly mental or physical.

THE CONCEPT OF A LIFE-SPAN

The concept within the models of a life-span from conception to death was handled efficiently by the contributors. The patients/clients in the studies included a newborn baby, an infant, and the remainder represented most of the decades of living (15, 22, 38, 41, 53, 67 and 86 years). The midwives' need for information about the prenatal care of the mother and the fact that the mother required extra information about contraception and family planning is tribute to the usefulness of the 'life-span' starting with conception.

The fact that the medical patient (Ch. 8) died at the age of 41 is a reminder that death can occur anywhere along the life-span but the effect on the survivors when the breadwinner dies in the prime of life, as in this instance, is likely to have greater repercussions. The contributors were well aware of the extra support needed by the patient's wife who not only lost her husband, but had recently moved to the city because of her husband's work. This is an example of the inter-relatedness of the life-span data and the biographical data which had implications for nursing.

The majority of a health visitor's clients are babies in family units and elderly people — those at each end of the life-span. However, while carrying out her study (Ch. 5) with the baby, the health visitor discusses how inclusion of 'dying' in the AL list directed her to consider occasions in health visiting when knowledge about death, dying and bereavement would be needed. She gave as examples, when there had been a still birth, a previous infant death in the family, and when there was anxiety about cot death. This highlights the interrelatedness of the life-span with the ALs and it was the end point of death on the life-span which originally persuaded us to include 'dying' in the list of ALs.

THE CONCEPT OF A DEPENDENT/INDEPENDENT CONTINUUM

The concept within the models of a dependence/independence continuum for each of the ALs was interpreted and used by the contributors, the postnatal baby (Ch. 6) being an example of dependence in most ALs because she had not yet acquired the necessary skills for independence. In comparison, the medical patient (Ch. 8) provided an example of a person who had achieved complete independence for all ALs, but who prior to his death was almost totally dependent on nurses for the carrying out of most ALs. The study of the patient who was unconscious from head injury (Ch. 11) is an example of a 38-year-old man who had previously been independent but was, during the period of data collection, unable to speak and could only move his arms and legs with help; he was therefore dependent for all ALs except breathing. On the other hand, the study of the elderly patient (Ch. 7) shows how a severely disabled woman maintained independence for as many activities as she could manage, but was nevertheless dependent for some aspects of personal cleansing and dressing and was totally dependent for the AL of mobilising.

FOCUS ON THE INDIVIDUAL

The focus on the individual in the models is an obvious starting point for individualising nursing. Assessment within

the AL framework encourages increased awareness of individuality because the many factors which influence the carrying out of the ALs are considered in the model. It was reassuring that the contributors had little difficulty in interpreting this aspect of the model reflected in the Patient Assessment Form; not one of the documents developed by them had sections for recording social, psychological, and cultural data because these were accepted as factors that influence the way in which each person carries out each AL. But the district nurses (Ch. 10) did discuss a stage in their thinking when they felt that they needed a separate heading 'economic factors'; yet they came to realise that this information could be documented at the AL of working and playing since most people work to earn an income.

THE MODEL OF LIVING

In the model of living (*The Elements of Nursing*, p. 21) we discussed other dimensions to be considered in relation to the ALs. These were preventing activities, comforting activities and seeking activities. It is obvious that readers do not find this part of the model useful and we intend to simplify the model (Fig. 2.1, p. 6) by removing this part in the next edition of *The Elements of Nursing*.

THE MODEL FOR NURSING

In the model for nursing (*The Elements of Nursing*, pp. 62, 63) we described four components of nursing:

- the AL component
- the preventing component
- the comforting component
- the dependent component.

Our stance now is that the preventing and comforting components are subsumed in the AL component and can therefore be omitted. We now believe that effective use of the Form identifies the independent part of the nurse's role as described in *The Elements of Nursing* (p. 10). But for the majority of nurses there are dependent and interdependent parts of their role which derive from medical/other prescription. It may well be that nurses would prefer to think of just two components of nursing:

- the AL component
- the medically/other prescribed component.

Reflecting on the inclusion of the process of nursing in the model we decided we should use the terms in current use — assessment, planning, implementation and evaluation when we were preparing the manuscript for *The Elements of Nursing*. However we are becoming increasingly critical of them. In many ways it is unfortunate that the words 'assessment' and 'evaluation' have been used for two phases of the process of nursing. The definition in the *Concise Oxford Dictionary* of the verb 'to assess' is 'estimate the *value* of' and the definition in *Collins National Dictionary* of the noun 'assessment' is '*evaluation* of merits'. To add to the confusion, the words are sometimes used interchangeably in the nursing literature and as a matter of fact in some languages there is no equivalent for 'assessment'. Even when writing *Learning to Use the Process of Nursing* we were apprehensive and wrote (p. 5), 'Some nurses are confused about assessing and evaluating; some of the skills used are common to both activities, but evaluating involves comparison against an objective — the stated patient outcome.'.

Another term which we consider adds to the confusion is 're-assessment'. Much of the 'nursing process' literature states that if at the stage of evaluation the goal has not been achieved then the cycle of the process should be repeated starting with reassessment. But is there such an activity as 'reassessment' when assessment is an ongoing activity? Also one has to remember that in the case of non-achievement of a goal the nurse may use her professional judgement and select an alternative nursing intervention to achieve the already stated patient goal.

Not only in national literature but at international level it has become almost a convention that the nursing process has four phases — assessment, planning, implementation and evaluation. We have no wish to cause any further confusion at this point by suggesting alternative terms. However, we suggest that it is useful to interpret assessment as collecting patient data by observing, interviewing, measuring and testing. The goal-setting part of planning can then be written in terms which are amenable to observing, interviewing, measuring and testing, and then for the evaluation phase one could observe, interview, measure or test to discover whether or not the stated goal was being or had been achieved.

Speaking generally, the assessment, planning and implementing phases of the process have received more attention than evaluation. Perhaps more emphasis should be placed on the fact that the process is dynamic, that evaluation is an ongoing activity interrelated with all phases of the process (*The Elements of Nursing*, Fig. 1.2). Perhaps the evaluation phase has been difficult because the goals have not been couched in terms which are amenable to evaluation. The discussion in the previous paragraph may help readers to acquire the necessary skills to evaluate nursing interventions effectively, and thereby to be accountable for the service which they render.

In this chapter we have mentioned the major points arising from the comments of the practising nurses who have described how they used the Roper/Logan/Tierney model for nursing (which incorporates the process of nursing) in nine different practice settings. We stated in the preface that our objective was to test our belief that the model could be used in a variety of health care settings. Readers will agree that the nine patient studies are positive on that point.

We also said that we considered the exercise to be an important development in linking theory and practice. According to the contributors the basic students had little difficulty in using the AL framework. This bodes well for the model as a means of using the same mode of thinking about nursing in the educational establishment and in the practice areas. We also think that this could be a means of reducing stress for students as they rotate through the obligatory clinical placements.

We cannot stress too strongly that we were impressed with the adequate information collected about patients'/clients' personal circumstances, family and home environment by using our very simple Patient Assessment Form. The way in which contributors used this information is evident in their written studies.

We were also impressed with the change in the contributed patient studies, from the usual descriptive style to that of minimum description and maximum tabulated information, and yet in every one of the studies the patient/client is presented as an individual person, with a family and particular home circumstances.

The contributors were positive about using the model and most said they would be interested in using it on a wider scale. But if there is to be efficient reliable documentation of nursing for every patient/client, then application of a practical model along with the phases of the process demands simple manageable documents. We hope that any nurses who use the *Patient Assessment Form and Nursing Plan*, presented in this chapter as a result of the exercise, will make known to us and other nurses, the pros and cons which they encounter. Both the Form and the Plan reflect our model for nursing, and if they can be improved by feedback, then so much the better. After all a model is only an artefact; it provides growing points for new ideas. And certainly we plan to continue to review the Roper/Logan/Tierney model for nursing.

Fig. 12.1 (pp. 181–184)
Patient Assessment Form and Nursing Plan
The first two pages of this four-page document comprise a revised edition of the original Patient Assessment Form which first appeared in *The Elements of Nursing* and was used by contributors to this book. Only minor changes have been made in the format for 'biographical and health data' (*page one*). The layout for recording data from 'assessment of ALs' has been changed: instead of an allocated space for each of the 12 ALs, the page has been left blank to allow the nurse to use the space to the best advantage for the particular patient (*page two*).

We have added to the Patient Assessment Form a two-page Nursing Plan. The first section (*page three*) makes provision for documentation of goals, nursing intervention and evaluation 'related to ALs'. The second section (*page four*) is for documentation of nursing intervention, goals and evaluation 'derived from medical/other prescription'.

This Patient Assessment Form and Nursing Plan is copyright and may not be reproduced in any form without the prior permission of the publishers (Churchill Livingstone, Robert Stevenson House, 1–3 Baxter's Place, Leith Walk, Edinburgh EH1 3AF).

Patient Assessment Form : Biographical and health data

Date of admission

Date of assessment

Nurse's signature

Surname   Forenames

Male ☐   Age ☐   Prefers to be addressed as

Female ☐   Date of birth _____

Single/Married/Widowed/Other

Address of usual residence

Type of accommodation
(incl. mode of entry
if relevant)

Family/Others at this residence

Next of kin   Name   Address

                     Relationship   Tel. no.

Significant others
(incl. relatives/dependents
visitors/helpers
neighbours)

Support services

Occupation

Religious beliefs and relevant practices

Significant life crises

Patient's perception of current health status

Family's perception of patient's health status

Reason for admission

Medical information (e.g. diagnosis, past history, allergies)

GP Address Tel. no.   Consultant Address Tel. no.

Plans for discharge

Patient Assessment Form: Assessment of ALs

Date

Activity of living AL	Usual routines: what he/she can and cannot do independently	Patient's problems: actual / potential (p)

Reminder of the 12 ALs

Maintaining a safe environment
Communicating
Breathing
Eating and drinking
Eliminating
Personal cleansing and dressing
Controlling body temperature
Mobilising
Working and playing
Expressing sexuality
Sleeping
Dying

Page two   *Roper, Logan, Tierney*   © Longman Group Limited 1983

Nursing Plan: Related to ALs

Goals	Nursing interventions related to ALs	Evaluation

Roper, Logan, Tierney

Nursing Plan: Derived from medical/other prescription

Nursing interventions derived from medical/other prescription	Goals	Evaluation

Other Notes

    Roper, Logan, Tierney

Appendix

The following summary charts from *The Elements of Nursing* were devised as an aide memoire at the end of discussion of each AL to help with collecting AL data. In addition to listing factors relevant in assessment they include patients' possible problems and the kind of nursing activities related to patients' problems with that AL.

Maintaining a safe environment

ASSESSMENT

Influencing factors
stage of development
physical factors
hearing
seeing
touching
tasting
smelling
dizziness
mobilising ability
mobility aids
psychological factors
intelligence
knowledge of and attitudes to
safety at home/work/play
road safety
smoking
handwashing
spread of infection
medicines/poisons
alcoholism
personality and temperament
awareness of danger
socio-economic factors
housing
social class
economic status

Standard of safety in the home
tidiness
flooring
water supply
heat and light supply
toilet facilities
storage of medicines/poisons
state of stairs/steps/paths
hygiene standards
fire precautions

Evidence of safety when working and playing
protective clothing
smoking habits
safety of equipment
safe use of equipment
safety of environment
safe behaviour

ANALYSIS OF DATA

IDENTIFICATION OF PATIENTS' PROBLEMS

Change of environment
unfamiliar environment
noise
nervousness
exposure to micro-organisms
exposure to hazards, such as oxygen
therapy

Change of routine
cleansing routines
taking medications

Change of mode
visual impairment/loss
aural impairment/loss
smelling and tasting
impairment/loss
mobilising impairment/loss
memory impairment/loss
reaction time impairment
psychological impairment

Dependence/independence in maintaining a safe environment
mental problems
physical problems

PLANNING

IMPLEMENTATION
of nursing activities such as

Orientating patient to new physical
environment

Matching of bed/chair to patient

Maintaining a quiet environment

Helping to decrease patients' anxiety

Liaising with domestic staff to maintain
hygiene standards

Practising/facilitating/encouraging
handwashing

Teaching patients and public about
maintaining a safe environment

Giving medications safely/keeping
drugs safely

Helping impaired patients to maintain a
safe environment

EVALUATION

Communicating

ASSESSMENT

Influencing factors
stage of development
physical factors
speaking
seeing
hearing
reading
writing
psychological factors
level of intelligence
extent of vocabulary
nervousness
prevailing mood
level of self-respect
sociocultural factors
native language
local vocabulary
accent/dialect
personal appearance/dress
touching
eye-contact
gesticulation
environmental factors
response to:
type/size of room
arrangement of chairs
background noise
light
room temperature
individual habit

Visual perception

Aural perception

Congruence of body and verbal language

Orientation
time of day
day of week
month of year

ANALYSIS OF DATA

IDENTIFICATION OF PATIENTS' PROBLEMS

Change of environment
unfamiliar people
unfamiliar place
unfamiliar language
unfamiliar activities
change of status and roles

Change in mode of communicating
impaired cognition
impaired/loss of sight
impaired/loss of hearing
impaired/loss of sensation
impaired/loss of mobility
impaired/loss of speech

Dependence/independence in communicating
cognitive problems
speaking problems
hearing problems
reading and writing problems
body language problems

Discomforts associated with communicating
pain
social embarrassment

PLANNING

IMPLEMENTATION
of nursing activities such as

Introducing patients to nurses and other patients

Talking with a purpose to patients and others

Establishing/maintaining/terminating nurse-patient relationships satisfactorily

Giving information clearly to patients and others

Teaching patients and others

Keeping patients orientated in time and place

Helping to prevent patients from feeling stigmatised

Communicating with:
deaf and hard of hearing patients
blind and visually-impaired patients
speech-impaired patients
cognitively-impaired patients
illiterate patients
immobile patients
breathless patients

Easing difficulty with speaking

Easing difficulty with seeing

Easing difficulty with hearing

Alleviating pain interfering with communicating

EVALUATION

Breathing

ASSESSMENT

Respiration and relationship to
 age
 weight
 pulse rate
 body temperature
 activity level
 emotional status
 colour of:
  skin
  mucous membrane
  nail bed

Character of breathing
 rate
 depth
 rhythm
 sound

Difficulty associated with breathing
 on inspiration/expiration
 on lying down
 on exertion

Cough (if present)
 when it occurs
 frequency
 what relieves it
 relationship to smoking
 sputum:
  amount
  colour
  odour

Smoking habits (if acquired)
 type of smoking:
  cigarette
  cigar
  pipe
 frequency
 tar content of tobacco
 reason for smoking
 intention to continue/give up
 relationship to present illness
 knowledge about adverse effects

Exposure to/knowledge of air pollution
 at home
 at work
 in neighbourhood

ANALYSIS OF DATA

IDENTIFICATION OF PATIENTS' PROBLEMS

Change of environment and routine

Change in breathing habit
 upper respiratory tract congestion
 excessive secretions
 bronchial spasms
 dyspnoea:
  interference with:
   speaking
   eating
   drinking
   working and playing
   mobilising
   sleeping
   expressing sexuality

Dependence/independence in breathing
 obstructed air passages
 oxygen insufficiency
 mechanical defect
 respiratory failure

Discomforts associated with breathing
 cough
 sputum
 haemoptysis
 allergy
 pain
 anxiety

Presence of
 artificial airway
 tracheostomy
 artificial ventilation equipment

Inability to give up/reduce smoking

PLANNING

IMPLEMENTATION
of nursing activities such as

Allaying anxiety associated with dyspnoea

Relieving dyspnoea

Administering oxygen

Maintaining an artificial airway

Maintaining tracheostomy toilet

Helping patient to expectorate sputum

Preventing/counteracting respiratory failure

Teaching and helping with breathing exercises

Alleviating discomforts associated with breathing

Assessing pain associated with breathing

Providing health education about:
 smoking
 room ventilation
 air pollution

EVALUATION

Eating and drinking

ASSESSMENT

Influencing factors
age and sex
height and weight
occupation and activity
state of mouth and teeth
proficiency in taking food and drink
emotional status
family traditions
sociocultural idiosyncrasies
religious commendations/
restrictions
finance available for food/drink
physical environment

Individual habits
timing and location of meals
quantity and quality of diet
consumption of alcohol
dietary likes and dislikes
deliberate restrictions/indulgences
company at mealtimes

Knowledge about/attitudes to
the effect of diet on health
obesity
alcoholism
food hygiene
disposal of food waste

Ability to procure food and fluid
facilities for growing food/procuring
water
choice and price of food/fluid
distance from home to shopping area
availability of transport
ability to carry shopping

Storage and cooking facilities
means of storage
means of cooking

Aids needed for independence
special utensils
mechanical aids
kitchen gadgets
special transport for shopping

Appetite for food/fluid

**Pain associated with eating and
drinking**
location/severity
type/duration

Discomforts
nausea/vomiting
indigestion/flatulence

ANALYSIS OF DATA

IDENTIFICATION OF PATIENTS' PROBLEMS

Change of environment and routine
timing of meals
serving of meals
pre- and post-meal activities
alteration in appetite
separation from mother

Dependence/independence
problems associated with physical
dependence
problems associated with emotional
dependence

Change in eating and drinking habits
modification of habitual food intake
modification of habitual fluid intake

Change in mode of eating and drinking
nasogastric feeding
gastrostomy feeding
intravenous feeding

**Discomforts associated with eating
and drinking**
stomatitis
nausea
vomiting
heartburn
flatulence
halitosis
pain
anxiety about investigations

PLANNING

IMPLEMENTATION
of nursing activities such as

Providing assistance necessary for
procuring/preparing food

Providing assistance/special
equipment necessary for eating and
drinking

Feeding by artificial routes

Maintaining an intravenous infusion

Assisting with planning and preparing
special diets

Teaching about special diets

Monitoring and recording food/fluid
intake

Preventing and controlling dehydration
and oedema

Assessing/alleviating pain associated
with eating/drinking

Alleviating discomforts associated with
eating/drinking

Providing health education about
nutrition and alcoholism

Controlling environmental factors
which affect preparation/eating/
disposal of foods and fluids

EVALUATION

Eliminating

ASSESSMENT

Urinary elimination
micturition frequency
urine output/fluid balance
appearance, smell, composition of
urine
discomforts associated with
micturition

Faecal elimination
defaecation frequency
factors altering frequency of
defaecation
amount, appearance, composition of
faeces
dietary habits, including fibre intake
measures taken to prevent
constipation
discomforts associated with
defaecation

Personal eliminating routine/habits
usual daily eliminating routine
type of toilet facilities available in
ward/home/work
habits regarding perineal toilet
habits regarding handwashing after
eliminating

**Dependence/independence in
eliminating**
degree of independence in
eliminating, related to age,
physical/mental/health
status, available toilet facilities
use of/need for special equipment/
appliances
history and nature of incontinence, if
relevant
details of catheter/stoma
management, if relevant

ANALYSIS OF DATA

IDENTIFICATION OF PATIENTS' PROBLEMS

Change of environment and routine
unfamiliar environment of hospital
unfamiliar routine of hospital life
lack of privacy in the ward

**Dependence/independence in
eliminating**
dependence due to:
limited mobility
confinement to bed
psychological disturbance

Change in urine and its elimination
anxiety about change in appearance
of urine
increased frequency of micturition
increased/decreased output of
urine
urinary incontinence
urinary catheterisation

Change in faeces and their elimination
anxiety about change in appearance
of faeces
increased frequency of defaecation:
diarrhoea
decreased frequency of defaecation:
constipation
inability to defaecate: impaction
faecal incontinence
ileostomy/colostomy

**Discomforts associated with
eliminating**
pain associated with micturition
pain associated with defaecation
anxiety associated with related
investigations

PLANNING

IMPLEMENTATION
of nursing activities such as

Providing opportunities, facilities,
privacy for eliminating

Giving assistance to dependent patients

Practising/facilitating/encouraging
handwashing

Ensuring safe disposal of excreta

Collecting and testing specimens of
urine/faeces

Monitoring and recording fluid balance

Catheterisation and catheter care

Preventing and treating constipation/
faecal impaction

Nursing a patient with diarrhoea

Nursing a patient with a stoma

Alleviating and preventing discomforts
associated with eliminating

Assessing and alleviating pain
associated with eliminating

Preparation of patients undergoing
investigations

Assisting/retraining the incontinent
patient

Teaching people about the AL of
eliminating

Teaching people how to prevent and
recognise related problems

EVALUATION

Personal cleansing and dressing

ASSESSMENT

Influencing factors
sex and stage of development
environment: fixed bath/shower;
piped hot/cold water
economic status; occupation climate;
cultural attitudes
individual habit

Skin
appearance: colour/bruising/scars;
turgid/wrinkled; dry/moist;
blemishes
areas of discontinuity: maceration;
athlete's foot; skin lesion/disease;
incision; pressure sores
degree of risk of pressure sores
bathing/showering: frequency; time
of day; aids needed/help required

Hands and nails
cleanliness; condition; abnormalities
evidence of type of occupation
handwashing routine/facilities

Hair
style, length, type: dry/greasy; dull/
shiny
presence of dandruff/nits
baldness
relationship to diet and health
hair washing routine/help required

Mouth and teeth
moistness/dryness of mouth/tongue
/lips
odour of breath
teeth: appearance; presence/
absence; plate, dentures/help
required; cleaning routine/help
required

Dress
style/colour/fashion
quality/newness of garments
quality/suitability of footwear
standard of cleanliness/odour
special clothing

Dressing
mobility problems
necessary modifications/help needed

ANALYSIS OF DATA

IDENTIFICATION OF PATIENTS' PROBLEMS

Change of environment and routine
unfamiliar ward routine
interference with daily routine
lessened decision making
lack of privacy

Change in mode of personal cleansing and dressing
imposed non-bathing
modification of clothing
wearing a prosthesis

Dependence/independence in personal cleansing and dressing
limited mobility
absence of limbs
involuntary movements
sensory deficits
unconsciousness
psychological disturbance
illness

Loss of skin continuity
incision
trauma
skin disease
pressure sores

Discomforts associated with personal cleansing and dressing
psychological discomfort
increased sweating

PLANNING

IMPLEMENTATION
of nursing activities such as

Providing opportunities, facilities, privacy
for continuance of patients' individual
habits

Giving assistance to dependent patients
without loss of their dignity

Providing opportunity for patients to
make decisions about their
personal cleansing and dressing

Using resources to help patients select
modified clothing and aids to
independence

Teaching patients and the public about
personal hygiene by, among other
methods, acting as a role model

Preparing patients' skin for operation

Carrying out wound dressing procedures
with aseptic technique

Monitoring patients at risk of
developing pressure sores

Preventing and treating pressure
sores

Treating infested patients

Helping patients who have an itching
skin

EVALUATION

Controlling body temperature

ASSESSMENT

Measurement of body temperature
> changes in body temperature over time
> relationship of ascertained temperature and changes to physiological, emotional, environmental and socio-economic factors
> ability to assist in controlling body temperature
> subjective feeling of being too warm/cold

Indicators of an abnormally high temperature
> flushed skin
> increased sweating
> increased pulse rate
> decreased urine output
> anorexia
> disorientation

Indicators of an abnormally low temperature
> pallor
> shivering
> decreased respiration rate/pulse/ BP
> lethargy
> impairment of consciousness

Risk of developing hypothermia

Knowledge of causes/prevention/ treatment of
> pyrexia
> heatstroke
> hypothermia

ANALYSIS OF DATA

IDENTIFICATION OF PATIENTS' PROBLEMS

Uncomfortable environmental temperature

Abnormally high body temperature

Abnormally low body temperature

PLANNING

IMPLEMENTATION
of nursing activities such as

Regulating environmental temperature

Measuring/recording body temperature

For a pyrexial patient
> preventing further increase of body temperature
> reducing body temperature to patient's normal level
> alleviating discomforts associated

For a hypothermic patient
> restoring body temperature to patient's normal level
> maintaining vital functions of the body

Prevention and early detection of hypothermia

Prevention of illness due to heat

EVALUATION

Mobilising

ASSESSMENT

Influencing factors
  developmental
  physical
  psychological
  environmental
  social

Mobilising habits
  at home/work/play

Musculoskeletal status
  adequacy of nervous and
    cardiopulmonary systems
  body posture and gait
  muscle strength, mass, tone
  range of movement in limbs, trunk,
    head and neck
  range of facial mobility
  joint movement and related stiffness/
    pain

**Dependence/independence in
mobilising**
  level of independence in the AL of
    mobilising
  mode of transport to work/school/
    shops
  aids needed for independent
    mobilising
  factors limiting independence

Knowledge and attitudes
  knowledge about the body's exercise
    needs
  attitude to physical handicap

ANALYSIS OF DATA

IDENTIFICATION OF PATIENTS' PROBLEMS

Change in mobilising routine

**Lack of specific knowledge about
mobilising routine**

Change in mobilising habit
  restricted mobility, including bedrest
  impairment of body or limb
    movement
  hyperactivity/hypoactivity
  physical handicap

Dependence in mobilising
  upper limb defect
  lower limb defect

Discomforts
  musculoskeletal discomforts
  therapeutic immobilising
    procedures
  pain
  social/economic and emotional
    discomforts

PLANNING

IMPLEMENTATION
of nursing activities such as

Giving assistance to patients with
  restricted mobility

Preventing/alleviating discomforts
  associated with reduced mobility

Assessing and alleviating pain
  associated with mobilising

Helping patients to accept and cope with
  the physical, socio-economic and
  psychological problems arising from
  restricted mobility

Lifting and moving patients

Teaching/supervising deep breathing
  exercises

Assisting with passive/active exercises

Providing/assisting with use of special
  equipment to aid mobilising

Restructuring the environment to
  maximise independence

Assisting/protecting the hyperactive/
  hypoactive patient

Planning, implementing and evaluating
  rehabilitation related to mobilising

Educating the public about physical
  handicap: implications/prevention

Educating the public about the body's
  exercise needs

Teaching people safe lifting techniques

EVALUATION

Working and playing

ASSESSMENT

Influencing factors
physical factors:
ability/disability
communicating ability
psychological factors:
intelligence
motivation
temperament and personality
traits
cultural and religious factors
climatic and environmental factors
economic factors

Routine regarding
time spent working/playing
place of working/playing
travel to place of working/playing
safety while working/playing
holidays from work/date of last one

Attitudes and habits regarding
punctuality and self-discipline
reliability and honesty
fulfilment/boredom
colleagues at work and play
sharing in group activities
earning and spending money

**Relationship between working/
playing and**
age and sex
emotional status
family circumstances
socio-economic status

Health status
effect of present illness on working/
playing

**Aids needed for independence in
working/playing**
special transport
special equipment

Knowledge and attitudes to
sick-leave from work
sickness benefit
safety at work/play
the importance of playing

ANALYSIS OF DATA

IDENTIFICATION OF PATIENTS' PROBLEMS

Change of environment and routine
change of working and playing
routines
absence from family groups
absence from work and play groups

**Dependence/independence in
working and playing**
congenital mental and/or physical
handicap
chronic disabling disease
impairment of the nervous system
mental illness
frailty

Change in working and playing habits
sensory deficits
physical disablement
physical disfigurement
change due to drug taking

**Discomforts associated with working
and playing**
boredom
lack of fresh air and exercise
economic hardship

PLANNING

IMPLEMENTATION
of nursing activities such as

Preventing boredom/providing
stimulation
playing/talking with patients
discussing with patient/parent/
guardian:
visiting/visitors
rooming-in
how the patients will occupy
themselves
enabling patients' activities to fit in to
treatment programme
helping patients to continue their
health habits/walking outside

Preventing loneliness
helping patients to benefit from
visitors
introducing patients to those with
similiar interests

Procuring aids to independence

Co-ordinating the contribution of:
occupational health service
Disablement Resettlement Officer
physiotherapists
occupational therapists
industrial therapists
speech therapists
social workers

Helping patients to return to, or change,
their working/playing habits

Helping patients with financial problems

EVALUATION

Expressing sexuality

ASSESSMENT

Stage of sexual development

Mode of expressing sexuality
in appearance, general behaviour, communication

Influencing factors
gender
stage of development
nature of relationship network
personal preference
social and family background

Effects of hospitalisation/disease/ disability
on sexual development
sexual relationships
sexual function
mode of expressing sexuality

Knowledge and attitudes about sex and reproduction
if relevant, history related to menstruation, contraception, pregnancy and parity
if relevant, detailed assessment of discomforts/dysfunction related to sexual organs/ function

ANALYSIS OF DATA

IDENTIFICATION OF PATIENTS' PROBLEMS

Anxiety/embarrassment about intimate procedures

Lack of privacy in the hospital ward

Restrictions on normal sexual development/activity imposed by hospitalisation

Sexual difficulties arising from
physical disease
physical disability
physical disfigurement

PLANNING

IMPLEMENTATION
of nursing activities such as

Preventing embarrassment/anxiety over intimate procedures

Providing maximum privacy for patients

Minimising disruption to established sexual habits/relationships during illness/hospitalisation

Ensuring opportunities for normal sexual development during long-term hospitalisation

Providing information about resuming/ restricting sexual activity after illness or surgery

Helping patients to cope with sexual difficulties

Preventing/alleviating discomforts associated with sexual function

Helping people to understand, develop and enjoy their sexuality

Health education about sex, reproduction, contraception, sexually transmitted diseases, sexual difficulties

EVALUATION

Sleeping

ASSESSMENT

Usual sleeping environment
bed/bedding/personal night attire
own/shared bed
own/shared bedroom
noise/quietness
hot/cold

Usual sleeping behaviour
work-shift/sleep pattern
time of going to bed
time of going to sleep
wakening during sleep/time of such
    waking
movement during sleep
snoring
time of wakening at end of sleep
    period
time of rising

**Patient's estimation of usual
sleeping**
good/bad sleeper
refreshed/unrefreshed on waking
mood on rising

Other factors influencing sleep
biological clock
daytime exercise
sleeping pills

Factors interfering with sleep
mood
worry, anxiety, apprehension
boredom
pain

Level of consciousness

ANALYSIS OF DATA

IDENTIFICATION OF PATIENTS' PROBLEMS

Change of environment and routine
bed, bedding, night attire
pre-sleep routine
posture
environmental temperature
noise
light
disturbance of circadian rhythm

Discomforts associated with sleeping
insomnia
    inability to get to sleep
    excessive wakefulness
    early morning waking
restlessness
cramp
pain

Impairment of consciousness
coma
convulsions

PLANNING

IMPLEMENTATION
of nursing activities such as

Facilitating continuation of pre-sleep
    routines

Ensuring comfortable environment for
    sleeping

Monitoring/recording sufficient/
    insufficient sleep

Preventing/alleviating factors
    interfering with sleep

Assessing and alleviating pain

Helping people to understand their sleep
    needs

Helping patients to cope with worries
    about sleeping

Safe administration, and monitoring
    effectiveness of sleeping pills

Health education about the hazards of
    sleeping pills

Care of an anaesthetised patient

Care of a comatose patient

Care of a convulsing patient

EVALUATION

Dying

ASSESSMENT

The person's
    physical status
    degree of pain
    discomforts
    degree of dependence/
        independence in all ALs
    awareness of the prognosis
    mood and behaviour
    fears and anxieties
    religion/beliefs about death and
        dying
    family and social circumstances
    wishes regarding care during
        terminal illness (including place
        of care, treatments, contact with
        family/others/chaplain)

The family's (significant others)
    knowledge of the prognosis
    understanding the implications of
        the prognosis
    reactions to this knowledge
    wishes regarding management of
        the terminal illness
    wish to contribute to care
    need for emotional support
    need for preparation for
        bereavement
    need for support in bereavement

ANALYSIS OF DATA

IDENTIFICATION OF PATIENTS' PROBLEMS

Physical problems associated with terminal illness
    pain
    other physical discomforts

Psychological problems in the terminal illness
    patient's problems
    relatives' problems

Problems associated with bereavement
    physical problems
    emotional problems

PLANNING

IMPLEMENTATION
of nursing activities such as

Helping the patient to die with dignity

Preventing suffering from pain in the terminal illness

Alleviating discomforts associated with all ALs

Providing companionship/preventing loneliness

Listening to anxieties/allaying fears and anxieties

Respecting as far as possible the patient's wishes

Providing opportunities and privacy for contact with loved ones

Providing information for relatives/ visitors

Providing emotional support for relatives/visitors

Preparing relatives for bereavement

Providing support for colleagues

Educating people about death, dying and bereavement

EVALUATION